W9-AOL-299

# People are already talking about *She-quel*

"Dr. Sherry breaks down all taboos about female anatomy in a way that makes you feel like you are talking to a trusted friend or a big sister. She gives you real, no nonsense answers to questions you might never have thought to ask. Even the embarrassing ones!"

—Reese Witherspoon, Academy Award-Winning Actress and Founder of the media production company, Hello Sunshine

"Dr. Sherry is my own personal advocate for holistic wellness and I love her. I am proud to have Dr. Sherry in my corner—not only as an expert and doctor but as a kind and compassionate champion for all women and children. I love knowing that—even if they are embarrassed to talk so openly with their own doctors—my sisters and friends can have access to the same life-changing information about their bodies, their female health, and their vaginas that I have had—and have a good laugh along the way. I wholeheartedly recommend Dr. Sherry's second book—*she-ology, the she-quel.*"

—Jennifer Garner, Actress and Co-Founder of Once Upon a Farm, a company dedicated to providing high-quality nutrition for children *everywhere*

"Dr. Sherry Ross is one of the brightest and smartest doctors we know. She has mastered her particular expertise, and women (and men) have benefited enormously from her knowledge. She has de-mystified so many 'taboo' subjects—bringing them into the forefront of her conversations with patients rather than having unanswered questions lurking in the darkness.

"As a couple, we feel that she is there for us at all the right times with just the right answers—even if it's not what we want to hear. A calm and truthful voice who is always trying to get to the root of the problem."

—Katharine McPhee, Actress, Singer, Songwriter and David Foster, Grammy Award-Winning Record Producer, Songwriter, and Composer

"I'll be the first to admit, I'm biased, but Dr. Sherry is my favorite gynecologist on the planet. She has been an amazing asset over the years, by helping me ease my hormonal self and keep it all together, as a career woman, mother, and wife. Dr. Sherry is truly one of the smartest and most amazing people I have ever met. I completely trust her with my life as well as that of my child, which she delivered. She is the wizard of gynecology and I want to share her with everyone I can! Do yourself a favor and read her book. You will be glad you did!"

—Debbie Metenopoulos, Host and Lifestyle Expert of Hallmark Channel's *Home & Family* show

"Dr. Sherry is a front-line warrior in the education of women of all types and ages. And I say that from personal experience as she has not only been my doctor, she has been my friend for nearly twenty-five years. She has walked the walk, accompanying me along my journey from pregnancy, dealing with my BRCA positive diagnosis, and the care and education of my teenage daughters and mother. She has championed and informed women in all aspects of health and wellness and continues to do so with this book. *She-quel* continues a life-changing conversation. Read this book and learn from the best!"

—Jennifer Salke, Head of Amazon Studios and Former President of NBC Entertainment

"Dr. Sherry is a marvel. She's brilliant and compassionate and no-nonsense. But mostly she believes passionately and unequivocally that women have a right and responsibility to understand their own bodies. So much of our own physiology is still shrouded in mystery, and Dr. Sherry will not accept that. With her first book, and now the sequel, she gives us explanations to experiences we've been conditioned not to ask about along with the tools to make our own physical (and emotional) lives easier. As a writer, a woman and mother of two, I'm so grateful her books exist."

—Sarah Treem, Writer, Producer, Playwright and co-creator and showrunner for the Golden Globe winning show *The Affair*

# she-ology the she-quel

## LET'S CONTINUE THE CONVERSATION

Sherry A. Ross, MD

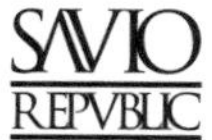

A SAVIO REPUBLIC BOOK
An Imprint of Post Hill Press

She-ology, The She-quel:
Let's Continue the Conversation
© 2020 by Sherry A. Ross, MD
All Rights Reserved

ISBN: 978-1-64293-180-8
ISBN (eBook): 978-1-64293-181-5

Illustrations by Ann-Marisa Wada
Interior design and composition, Greg Johnson, Textbook Perfect

The information and advice herein is not intended to replace the services of trained health professionals or be a substitute for individual medical advice. You are advised to consult your health professional with regard to matters related to your health, and in particular regarding matters that may require diagnosis or medical attention.

No part of this book may be reproduced, stored in a retrieval system, or transmitted by any means without the written permission of the author and publisher.

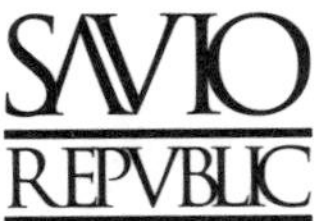


posthillpress.com
New York • Nashville
Published in the United States of America

*To my father,*
*who gave me strength, wisdom, and a sense of humor,*
*and who taught me to persevere.*

*To my mother,*
*who remains for me a beacon of hope,*
*and a constant source of love and inspiration.*

*To my wife and sons,*
*who keep my heart full of endless love, laughter,*
*and possibilities each and every day.*

# TABLE OF CONTENTS

# FOREWORD

## Julia Ormond

In my twenties, my boyfriend was a gynecologist. For fun, I would call him at work and ask *if he could chat, or if he had his hands full.* He'd wait patiently on the phone for me to stop laughing at my own joke. Friends couldn't fathom how I could trust a sexual relationship with him. They wondered: Wasn't he screwed up from looking at women's 'bits' all day? Was he screwed up to begin with? Was he perversely obsessed with vaginas? And why on earth would someone frigging decide on gynecology as their chosen path? It seemed such a narrow, rather dubious choice of career. In fact, he was one of the kindest souls I'd ever met. Not only was he a loving boyfriend, he set the bar high for whoever would become my gynecologist.

Fortunately, I found that bar met by Sheryl Ross, my gynecologist now for over a decade. By sharing her wisdom and compassion, Dr. Sherry has helped empower me to take care of my sexual health and myself as a woman. In doing so, I have found a greater sense of wholeness, and I am thrilled that she is putting pen to paper and sharing that wisdom more widely.

## She-ology the Shequel

It's hard not to have deep respect for someone who brings new human beings into the world for a living, who habitually puts parent and, I'm sure, child instantly at ease. Los Angeles is a diverse city, so as a "local" one has access to phenomenal people of every expertise—one of those people being Dr. Sherry, whom I'm both lucky and privileged to have found. Not only has she the smarts, experience, and empathy I believe necessary for someone in her profession, she can distill the most complicated and overwhelming information in a way that always makes me feel supported and at ease. I would encourage any and everyone to be guided by her.

In particular, Dr. Sherry has informed me by debunking the taboos around female sexuality that I had unconsciously pandered to. She eschewed nicknames for those "private bits," while gently, matter-of-factly providing answers and explanations to my concerns. Without ever lecturing or preaching, she erased my awkwardness and sloughed away the mystery I'd unknowingly cloaked around female sexual health.

Until meeting Dr. Sherry I'd always had a lingering anxiety about my sexual health, which led to an unconscious disconnect with my body—manifesting in my crass jokes and obligatory exclamations of "Ew!" in my first visits. Dr. Sherry countered by helping me to understand that my disconnect was antithetical to my sexual health, and, therefore, my *whole health*. It not only complicated healing; it created denial around preventative health.

I know now, at fifty-four, that it just won't do to feel "Ew" about any part of myself. Getting to the other side of that paradigm helped me to integrate and take back what was mine to begin with, but had seemed in service of others. Integrating my sexual parts, not as separate pieces but part of my whole, has been a door to profoundly transformative personal acceptance and growth. Equally profound is that this woman, Dr. Sherry, likely doesn't know how key she has been in my transformation. For that reason I'm grateful to have been asked to contribute to her book, and grateful to speak, as a patient, about how she has affected my life and my path. I'm honored to be witness to her unique blend of human power and insight into the care and culture of women.

From a very early age, a woman's private parts are, culturally, a mystery. This is expressed even in our design of public restrooms, where common male bonding occurs at the urinal. Boys are socially required to be familiar with their genitalia—in public, no less.

Women (and girls), on the other hand, pee in private. Because our sexual areas are, to an extent, internal, we are moved to maintain the mystery rather than question and challenge it. As a girl, I specifically remember wondering if "mine" were like other girls'. Of course, I was too embarrassed to ask anyone. (Sorry, Mum and Dad, but had porn been as easily accessible when I was going through puberty as it is today, I'm sure I'd have turned to it in search of that visual context, which would only have served to heighten my anxiety about my own body.) For far too long I had no idea if I was even normal. That "not knowing" put me at a disadvantage in my relationship to sex and my sense of self. As a girl I didn't feel comfortable asking my girlfriends if they felt the same way about their bodies I felt about mine, because I didn't want to solicit the habitual "Ew" response back. I wish I'd had this book to turn to. In lieu of that, I am grateful that I'll be able to hand it to my daughter.

Part of our development from girls to women is to look for ourselves in others—to search for role models. As a child, I looked to my mother. At puberty I looked to older girls. Now, as a mother and smack in the middle of menopause, I both seek and find affirmation in nature itself, finally feeling in sync with the cycles of the moon and seas and tides. I've experienced a greater connection to my body, largely through how I can feel when I'm sexually aroused. I find my growing appreciation of and respect for nature mirrored in my older self.

I wish for a world in which there is no one definition for normal, rather a recognition and celebration of depth and diversity. With this book, we may all have Dr. Sherry in our lives to remind us to celebrate, to anchor us, liberate us, and offset the relentless messaging to conform to boring clichés that reduce us and slow our strides, regardless of our sexual orientation. To this end, Dr. Sherry has made me a wiser woman. Perhaps she is birthing wise *people* as well as babies.

# INTRODUCTION

With She-ology 2.0, the vagina revolution continues!

In writing my first book *She-ology: The Definitive Guide to Women's Intimate Health. Period,* I not only wanted to answer the most common questions that women have about their vaginas—and are, unfortunately, too embarrassed to ask their health care providers—I wanted to address the cultural taboos and sensationalized aspects of that most amazing and often mystifying female organ.

Women want answers! So, even though I sought to include as many answers to as many questions that women have about their vaginas and their selves, since *She-ology* was published, I have received countless emails from women all over the world with questions about topics not covered in *She-ology*.

For example, one such topic had to do with conversations I have every day with women who come to me because they are having sex for the first time in *years*—for whatever reason; divorce, separation, abstinence—or they are in menopause and suddenly finding that sex is painful, or they're experiencing vaginal difficulties due to breast cancer recovery. For many of those women, the problem was a collapsed vagina, which led to a lengthy chapter called—what else—"The Collapsed V."

However, beyond the necessity to include topics that weren't in *She-1,* and despite knowing how difficult it is for women (and men) to even say the word vagina—let alone talk about its care and feeding—I was shocked at how resistant the mainstream media was in dealing with the content of She-ology!

This resistance became apparent during one of the first stops on my book promotion tour—and one of the highlights of that tour—an appearance on *The Rachel Ray Show.*

Now, I've always loved Rachel Ray. She is a vibrant example of a celebrity who has remained true to herself. So I was excited to talk with her about issues in the book related to PMS, menopause, and the clitoris—a medical term, mind you, as is the word *vagina*—but, just as I was readying myself for the taping, I was approached by the show's producer. I was reminded by her to be prudent in using the word "vagina," since it was, after all, "network TV." Also, I wasn't allowed to say the word "clitoris." To be fair, those precautions were dictated by the network and not by Rachel and her producers, but, even so, I couldn't help but think: *What kind of world do we live in where we can't use medical terms to describe a woman's genitalia?*

Not one to be deterred, especially on my mission to spread the gospel of the vagina, I used a variety of code names for vagina, names like vajayjay and happy valley. I even asked Rachel what she called hers. She responded by looking like a deer in headlights—apparently no one had ever asked her that question—but she quickly recovered and answered, "I don't call it anything."

The truth is that 40 percent of all women use code names in referring to their vaginas! One study of a thousand women showed that number to be as high as 65 percent, which is why

I remain on a mission to reclaim that word. Vagina. (I can only wonder what amusing little child-friendly name senate conservatives are using for the word "vagina" when talking about health care and contraception for women. *Oh, wait, they don't seem to be talking about it at all,* which is another reason why we need to take up the conversation about vaginas and their care and *importance.*)

If women and men can't even say the word vagina, how are we to have a dialogue about it?

Here in *She-ology 2.0,* I continue the dialogue begun in my first book. Both books are meant for women with vaginas, women or men who are in transition to having vaginas, and those of you who love someone with a vagina (I think that just about covers all people who ought to be concerned about vaginas). They're meant for anyone—female or male—and anyone who identifies as straight, gay, transgender, queer, inter-sex, or gender-neutral. These books are for *you.*

As a doctor and as a woman, I feel strongly obliged to provide women with information that may empower them to have conversations about their bodies and take control of their health and well-being. Every day, I take that obligation seriously in my practice, as well as in the articles I write and in the leadership opportunities I have been afforded.

Some would say that I have an agenda. Some would even call me The Vagina Whisperer. And that is true! I want to further this vagina revolution in order to create cultural change and a grass roots movement in preserving the well-being of all women.

That movement begins with informing young women about their bodies—especially their vaginas—and helping them to use their voices to ensure that they get the care they need. It seems that, overnight, I have begun to do gynecologic exams on young women that I *delivered*—talk about feeling one's age—and my first responsibility is to help them feel as comfortable as possible. Once their legs are in the stirrups, I pull out a mirror in order to give them a "show and tell" moment. As savvy as some of these young women are, I'd say that 99 percent of them have not looked at their own vagina and vulva. It's not difficult to gain their undivided attention as I go over every part of their genitalia. Many are shocked to see where urine comes from and glad to locate their clitoris. In fact, I encourage them to get to know their clitoris, and not to feel shame in learning how to masturbate, as chances are their first sexual encounters will not involve someone who knows how to sexually please them. I'm old enough to remember song lyrics along the line of "you can't please everyone, so you've got to please yourself." It kind of takes on new meaning in this context, don't you think?

As for you mothers (or caregivers) of daughters, it's not just about having "the talk"—meaning that one big talk about menstruation or sexual intercourse—it's about having *many* talks about their developing bodies and overall health. Before you start talking about sexuality and sexual behavior, you have to create an environment in which your daughter feels comfortable discussing other sensitive (age-appropriate) topics, such as body image, puberty, nutrition, alcohol, and drug use.

When young girls learn about their body parts—"Here is my nose, my ears, my belly button"—they need to learn and use the word vagina as well, in order to become comfortable with their own anatomy. If a girl only knows a cute code name for her vagina, the needle will not move in the right direction of the vagina narrative.

## Introduction

Girls need role models in initiating the often-sensitive conversations about sexuality, health, and wellness. Without those role models, they'll look to other resources, such as social media, porn, and websites promoting idealistic, unattainable, and unhealthy models of sex and body image, which only serve to damage one's self-worth.

My goal in speaking to women of all ages is to change the narrative on how women see and take care of their bodies and, more specifically, their vaginas. I'd like to enlist your help in doing so.

Have a conversation in the next few days with a girlfriend, a family member, your mother, daughter, or sister and use the word vagina, just once. Start a dialogue. Ask a question. Share your concerns. And look at it this way: one of those women's lives may depend on it.

As Ruth Bader Ginsberg so famously said, "Real change, enduring change happens one step at a time."

The Vagina Revolution continues, a revolution essential for women in embracing their sexuality, their identity, and their sense of selves.

*Vive la révolution—part deux!*

***—Dr. Sherry***

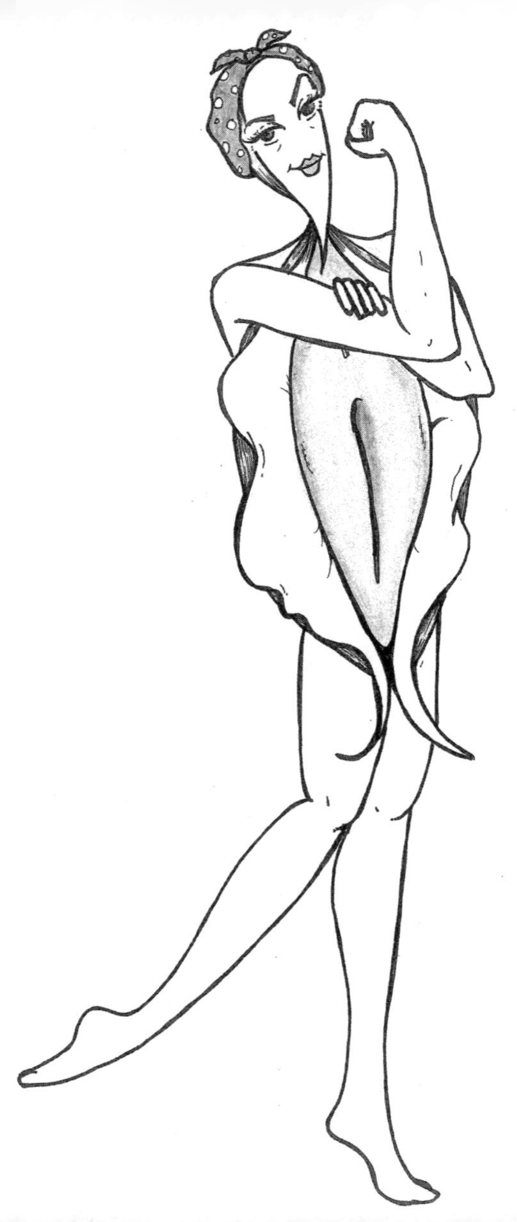

# CHAPTER 1
# confident

"Before I start, I feel obliged to come clean. I'm a health nut—or, put another way, I'm hell-bent on forestalling that which Mother Nature has in store for me and y'all. Supplementing my cocktail of determination with a healthy dash of neurosis, I have set my sites on things controllable that, *en masse*, qualify as 'Preventative Medicine.' It's not that I believe I can avoid the grim reaper forever; it's that my bucket list is long and growing, and I refuse to leave a whole lotta boxes unchecked....

Wading into the nature vs. nurture argument, I don't think I arrived on Mother Earth wired to eat coconut oil and green shakes. On the contrary, I grew up on a healthy diet (all in the eyes of the beholder at the time) of fried pork chops, sweet tea, and anything they could pour white sauce on. Heck, we even played in the fog spewing out the back of the DDT truck that careened down our street to protect us from the army of mosquitos with whom we shared our small Mississippi town.

All that came to a screeching halt when judgment day arrived (a.k.a. my mama was diagnosed with ovarian cancer after decades of no exercise, cigarettes, and diet cokes). Nine years in and out and back in hospitals in numerous states sobered me up really quickly. Suddenly, the grease that resided on the bottom of the to-go bag was a ticket to the ECU, not taste bud heaven. It was too late for my mama (she succumbed to an ailment that, no doubt, was not helped by her life choices), but not too late for me and my kids. A front row seat where I witnessed the 'effect' of the 'cause' was enough for me. My life changed on a dime.

Committed and determined to help my body and not hurt it, I made a conscious effort to harvest a lifestyle and choices based on new information, new alternatives, 'must dos' and 'can't haves.' The result was resurgence in health and a sense of well-being from foot to V to head!

With so many environmental toxins, harmful food additives, and GMOs swarming our grocery stores and restaurants, we have to be ever mindful in our own personal education. I have learned to question not only my food sources and the indecipherable ingredients in supposedly 'healthy' products, but even my educators, doctors, and supposed experts get a once-over before I follow them blindly. If what I'm hearing doesn't make sense or resonate for me, I look further. All of us must take responsibility for the quality of life that we wish upon ourselves, or else we will be part of the problem, not part of the solution.

Dr. Sherry's chapter, 'Confident V,' provides the launch pad for the kind of life I fight every day to live. I have little doubt that you'll find what you need to know about maintaining not only a confident V, but also a confident, healthy, and present self. ”

—**Sela Ward** Actress, Author, Producer

# Confident V

Here we are, the point of this book: to empower you to know and love your body and your vagina, which will, in turn, help you to fully love and appreciate and care for yourself. When that is accomplished, what you wind up with is the healthiest and happiest life possible. When you take care of yourself, when you become your own health advocate, you take control of your own life. It's not selfish. Think of it this way: When the airline attendant does her requisite emergency spiel at the beginning of a trip, she includes a demonstration of how to properly use the oxygen masks. Notice that she always says to put a mask on *yourself* before you try to assist another passenger, specifically the small child traveling with you. Think about it. If you don't take care and receive life-sustaining oxygen first, you are of no use to anyone, leastways yourself!

If only taking care of oneself in life were as simple as putting on that oxygen mask. Truth is there's so much information, misinformation, and confusion about women's health that it's hard to know where exactly to begin your self-health advocacy. I hear the same concerns from many different women.

*I'm so confused by all the new data about mammograms! How often do I get them?*

*When should I start bone density testing?*

*How do I maintain a healthy vagina?*

What I've compiled here are the answers to many and more of those questions, along with a guide to taking control of your preventative healthcare, and, in doing so, your life. Confident V, you are on!

## Confidence Via Lifestyle

Statistics tell us that the average woman will live to be eighty-one. Despite this good news, half of all adults struggle with one or more chronic diseases. In 2018, seven of the top ten causes of death were from chronic diseases, with almost half of those deaths attributable to the top two on the list—heart disease and cancer (breast and colon topping the cancer subset). From all the pink merchandising, one would think otherwise, but heart disease is the leading cause of death among women throughout the world. As far as those other chronic diseases are concerned, a recent study showed that 70 to 80 percent of them—including cardiovascular disease, diabetes, obesity, arthritis, and even some cancers—are caused by lifestyle.

Life. Style. Meaning that, in changing one's lifestyle, one may indeed alter one's health trajectory. So how can we live longer with a better quality of life? Read on!

## Four Essential Strategies to Maximizing Your Health

1. **Diet:** I've driven this one home before, but I can't stress enough the value of a healthy diet. A well-balanced plant-based diet with the consumption of "good" fats (meaning mono and polyunsaturated fats), limited intake of red meat and high-fat dairy and the elimination (or near elimination) of processed foods will promote healthy aging and reduce your risk of cardiovascular disease and breast cancer. The Mediterranean diet is a perfect model to follow in helping to avoid those two most common causes of death in women—heart disease and breast cancer. By modifying your diet, you can reduce your risk of obesity,

which affects more than one third of people in the United States and is a proven factor in an increased risk of heart disease, high blood pressure, Type-2 diabetes, arthritis-related disability, and some cancers. Obesity is at an all-time high affecting four of ten US women. Ideally, you want to keep your BMI (body mass index) under twenty-five for optimal health.

However, there has been a lot of attention on another point of view, regarding diet, BMI numbers, and obesity, termed *the obesity paradox*—which supports the opinion of grandmothers down the ages that having a few extra pounds actually prevents illness and other diseases long associated with a BMI over 30. The obesity paradox addresses the question: does weighing a few extra pounds actually help you fight disease, live longer, and make you healthier? My colleague and friend, nutrition expert, and therapist Elyse Resch, co-author of *Intuitive Eating and The Intuitive Eating Workbook,* seems to think so.

I asked Elyse to weigh in on the issues, and this is what she told me:

> *"We are constantly bombarded by messages from magazines, television, social media, etc. about what we should eat and how we should look. Those external messages often serve to make us doubt our inner wisdom. But your best source of information comes from that private place within you that knows when you're hungry and full, what meals are satisfying, and how your body feels. Grab your power and assert your autonomy—it's a sign of your mental health! Speak up for what you believe is best for you.*

*"Start by rejecting diet culture. You can't fool Mother Nature! Studies show that diets are doomed for failure—95 percent of people who go on diets gain the weight back, and two thirds of them gain even more weight. Why make yourself miserable by pursuing a path that's destined to make you feel defeated and ruin your self-esteem?*

*"Instead, treat your body with respect, regardless of your size or shape. Stop bashing your body and judging or comparing yourself to others. Fight weight stigma!"*

2. **Exercise:** Regular exercise can reduce every major chronic disease, specifically those diseases worsened by obesity. Walking at least thirty minutes a day, at least five times a week is excellent for overall good health and reduces your risk of cardiovascular death and breast cancer. As per the Department of Health and Human Services, "A minimum of 150 minutes of moderate aerobic activity or 75 minutes of vigorous aerobic activity a week, or a combination of moderate and vigorous activity is recommended for most healthy adults." Physical activity helps to increase lean muscle mass, strengthen the immune system, and promote mental and emotional well-being. *Aerobic* exercise is the most efficient way of getting your heart working at optimal levels. Even walking regularly can reduce blood pressure. Some love the challenge of keeping track of their steps with any one of the great new athletic devices and apps available—myself included. I find that having the goal in mind of 10,000 steps daily keeps me accountable to my exercise resolution. And with accountability comes success.

3. **Limit alcohol consumption:** We've known that alcohol consumption increases one's risk of heart disease, liver disease, high blood pressure, diabetes, and colorectal cancer, but now we can add breast cancer to those negative effects. It has been found that having *two or more drinks a day* increases the chance of developing breast cancer as much as 41 percent. Even moderate alcohol intake—defined by 1.5 ounces of hard liquor or a five-ounce glass of wine daily—slightly increases your risk of breast cancer. If you drink moderate amounts of alcohol, it's recommended to take 600mcg of folate to counteract (to some degree) alcohol's negative effects.
4. **Quit smoking:** The physical and emotional effects of smoking have been known for years. Quitting may be the single best thing you can do to avoid a variety of medical illness (heart disease, high blood pressure, and lung cancer, to name a few) and increase your life expectancy. Lung cancer caused by smoking is the leading preventable cause of cancer.

We have all heard the saying, "You are what you eat." I might make the adjustment that when it comes to our overall health, "We are how we live." Being realistic in your health care resolutions and keeping your goals as simple as possible will make you more likely to succeed at a healthy *lifestyle,* which should also include more than a few ounces worth of prevention in the form of screenings and exams. According the American College of Obstetrics and Gynecology, yearly well-woman exams throughout your life is the best time to connect with your healthcare providers for screening, evaluations, counseling, and immunizations on the basis of age and risk factors.

## Screenings and Exams Through the Decades

### *Teen Years*

The Human Papilloma Virus (HPV) vaccine is recommended at eleven to twelve years of age for both *girls and boys*. The reason for this early screening is to make certain you've been vaccinated *before* exposure to the virus, since HPV is the most common sexually transmitted infection, affecting 75–80 percent of men and women. There are around one hundred types of HPV carrying varied risks, the highest of which, known as 16 and 18, are associated with abnormal Pap smears and cervical cancer. Low risk HPV types are often associated with benign warts, and some types never physically express themselves. Your risk of exposure is directly related to the number of sexual partners you've had. More partners, greater risk. The latest and greatest Gardasil-9 vaccine is found to prevent 90 percent of cervical cancers caused by the most common types of HPV. And, in case you missed getting this lifesaving vaccine in your teens, the FDA has recently approved it up to age forty-five.

### *Your Twenties*

Twenty-one is the beginning of a whole new chapter for many women. It's also at about this age that women ought to begin routine annual pelvic examinations. The importance of birth control and safe sex is a major topic for most twenty-somethings, so annual well-woman visits with your OB-GYN or health care provider are important not only for your general physical health, but your mental well-being. Sexually active women should be screened for sexually transmitted infections (STIs)—including chlamydia and gonorrhea—yearly, after unprotected sex, or in between new partners. Of course, if you've left your teens without an HPV vaccine, it's now essential to remedy that. HIV testing needs to be done yearly as long as you remain sexually active with different partners (or your partner remains sexually active outside of your relationship).

As a reminder, safe sex means using a condom during vaginal or anal intercourse and oral sex (during which dental dams are used to protect the throat from HPV). And, if there isn't a dental dam in grabbing distance, plastic wrap or a cut condom will do the trick.

Cervical cancer screening begins at twenty-one and is repeated every three years thereafter. For women at low risk, Pap smears can be done every three years and HPV testing done every five if both tests are negative.

Timely topics to discuss with your health care provider may include period problems, cramps, PMS, painful sex, and any other concerns that arise.

### *Your Thirties*

If you've had normal Pap smear screenings throughout your twenties (and continue to do so), then you can combine your Pap smear along with an HPV test every three years.

Women under the age of thirty with a low risk strain of HPV will most likely have normal Pap smears in the future without any treatment. HPV in this age group tends to go away on its own. However, women aged thirty to sixty-five with a HPV of the high risk type are more likely to develop dysplasia or pre-cancer cells in following years, even with a normal Pap smear. If you have a history of abnormal Pap smears, you'll need screenings more often, since HPV is the direct link to those abnormal smears and increases the risk of cervical cancer.

The discussion of fertility and family planning should take a front seat in one's early thirties. It's a good time to ask yourself the following questions: How many children do I want? Am I willing to get pregnant without having a partner? How important is it to have my own biological child?

If you are single and you're not even thinking about future fertility, it may be time to have a conversation about egg freezing. The best candidates for egg freezing are women between the ages of thirty-one and thirty-eight who are delaying pregnancy by at least two years. For this age group, the success rate of a live birth with either frozen eggs or frozen embryos is 40 to 50 percent.

You may have to be the one to start this conversation with your health care provider in order to make plans for a possible future family, since many health care providers do not have the time or knowledge to help in future family planning. In any event, you don't ever want to look back when it's too late and say to yourself: *I wish I had been proactive in planning for my family.*

Breast cancer prevention begins in your thirties and lasts through most of your life. The routine of a healthy colorful diet, limited alcohol intake, regular exercise, weight control, and adequate levels of vitamin D is a routine that begins early in this decade and should last a lifetime.

BRCA1 and BRCA2 are precarious genetic mutations for which you may be tested around this time. Certain family histories put you at risk for these particular mutations associated with early breast and ovarian cancers. If you test positive for BRCA1 or BRCA2, you might be a candidate for an elective bilateral mastectomy and prophylactic oophorectomy (the removal of healthy ovaries in women who have an elevated risk for ovarian cancer) once you are done having children or by the age of thirty-five.

### *Your Forties*

Breast cancer affects one in eight women yearly, so early detection is key, which means that mammograms—still the best form of screening—begin at age forty and continue every year (or two) depending on your family history and risk factors. Certain factors undoubtedly create higher risk. These factors need to be considered by you and your healthcare provider on an individual basis. They include:

* Number of first-degree relatives with breast cancer
* Women who had their first menstrual period before age twelve
* Women who had their first pregnancy after age thirty or women who have never had a full-term pregnancy
* Number of previous breast biopsies
* Women who have already had breast cancer
* Presence of atypical hyperplasia
* Mammographic breast density
* Excessive alcohol consumption
* BMI greater than 30
* Physical inactivity

Become actively involved in your own breast health by educating yourself about your own personal risk factors. Age is no longer the only factor to take into account, so be informed. Champion your breast; champion your vagina...or vice versa!

As the leading cause of death in women, heart disease claims one in three women, which is why heart health screening is so important. Have a yearly cholesterol screening/ lipid profile and discuss with your internist whether an EKG or Stress Echocardiogram might also be necessary. Standard procedure at your yearly checkups ought to include checking blood pressure and fasting glucose levels, along with that most feared of procedures...*the weigh-ins.* Yes, this is all vital in looking out for hypertension, diabetes, and heart disease.

Unfortunately, there are no real tried-and-true screenings for ovarian cancer, a highly lethal cancer that tends to be diagnosed in late stages, since symptoms are slow to occur. That said, women at high risk for this disease, including those with a family history or those who have tested positive for BRCA1 and 2 mutations, Ashkenazi women with a single family member with breast cancer or ovarian before age fifty, ought to consider having a transvaginal pelvic ultrasound and CA-125 blood test every six to twelve months along with a pelvic examination.

Melanoma and other skin cancers can be detected by a dermatologist, which means a yearly "mole check" for most of us. A good dermatologist can tell the difference between a beauty mark and an abnormal skin change.

### *Your Fifties*

Osteoporosis is a disease in which bones become brittle, weak, and fragile, causing a decrease in quality and strength and ultimately leading to fractures and breaks. Women are *five times more likely* to develop osteoporosis than men, and the only way to tell if you have osteoporosis is through a bone density screening, which involves a type of X-ray that measures the thickness and density of bone. These screenings can begin in your fifties, depending on your risk factors. High risk factors for women include:

* Menopause
* Smoking history
* Excessive alcohol intake
* Family history of osteoporosis
* Steroid use
* Previous fractures

If you seem not to be at high risk, bone density testing can start at sixty-five.

Colon cancer, the second most common cancer to strike women (behind lung and ahead of breast), is actually in a 2–3 percent decline due to a rise in screenings and the adoption of better lifestyle choices over the past fifteen years. Early detection does save lives, so have that baseline colonoscopy at fifty (consider it a healthful birthday present) and continue those screenings every ten years. Yearly fecal occult blood testing is recommended in between colonoscopies.

Lung cancer screenings begin at around fifty-five. For women with a history of smoking, even if you are a reformed smoker and have quit in the past fifteen years, a low dose CAT scan screening ought to be performed annually. Early detection means a better chance of survival.

### *Your Sixties and Beyond*

Good news. After coming this far, you may actually stop cervical cancer screenings beyond age sixty-five, if you do not have a history of moderate or severe dysplasia or cancer, and if you've had either three negative Pap tests results in a row or two negative co-test results in a row within the past ten years (with the most recent test in the past five years). Women who have had a hysterectomy may still need screenings, depending on the reason for the hysterectomy and whether they've had a history of moderate or severe dysplasia.

For those women who haven't already begun bone density testing, now's the time to start. A repeat every two years is recommended for those at low risk.

Above and beyond and along with all this prevention and screening, regular visits to your general doctor or internist are important for your general health and well-being.

## Vitamins and Supplements

To take, or not to take, that is the question.

Truthfully, the best way to get your daily, required doses of vitamins, minerals, and antioxidants is through a well-balanced and colorful diet. The problem is that the average diet often leaves gaps in those daily nutritional needs, preventing your body from functioning at its optimal capacity. Therefore, a complete multi-vitamin may serve as the best policy to ensure that you're not missing out in your diet.

During pregnancy, breastfeeding, and certain medical conditions, additional vitamins are often called upon to meet the body's requirement for extra nutrients. Women who are trying to become pregnant need additional folic acid, while pregnant women need to supplement with certain vitamins and minerals such as calcium, iron, vitamins D, and B-complex. Best to add Omega-3 fatty acids as well. A good prenatal vitamin will have all the extra vitamins and minerals that your body will need during this hypermetabolic time.

Although supplementing your diet is important, vitamins can be harmful in mega doses or doses beyond the recommended daily allowance. Side effects from supplement/vitamin overdoses can range from mild, and include stomach upset, diarrhea, constipation, nausea, and vomiting, to severe, involving kidney stones, anemia, birth defects, liver damage, or other organ impairment.

If you are taking aspirin, blood thinners, steroids, or heart and immune-suppressing medication, ask your health care provider if vitamin supplements are safe. Vitamins can also potentially cause excessive bleeding and other complications during surgery.

Pay attention to what exactly you're taking. Remember that, when a product is described as "natural," it doesn't necessarily mean that it is safe for *you*, or that it is without side effects. And always find your vitamins and supplements from a reputable source. That "cheap" online company across the globe may not necessarily be the place to order something you put in your body daily.

For women over fifty, bones, heart, brain, and breast health are leading concerns. Be proactive with vitamins and minerals that are key in regard to these.

## A Personal Journey to a Confident V

Like many of you, I have my certain group of BFFs, those girlfriends with whom I would get together for weekly dinners, happy hours, or brunches during which the wine, Bloody Marys, Margaritas, and "light" beers accompanied lively (and livelier as the meals went on) conversations around relationships, kids, financial woes, and, yes, gossip—contrary to popular belief, doctors are definitely not immune to gossip. But, as a doctor, I always felt somewhat guilty the morning after in recalling the number of drinks I'd consumed, knowing full well that the recommended allowance for optimal health was two to three...*weekly*. After those get-togethers, my night's sleep would suffer interruptions, during which I would imagine, in full color detail, the damage I was doing to my liver and how I was increasing my risk of breast cancer, high blood pressure, and a host of other distressing medical conditions.

See, the thing is, although my driver's license reminded me that I was over fifty, I still *felt* like I was in my twenties. Despite that feeling, I knew that I had to be more mindful of the way I was walking through my life, which meant suggesting to my friends that our weekly get-togethers needed to focus on healthier living. My friends—most of them my age—understood, even though we didn't *really* want to talk about it. Talking about it made aging a reality; it made our birthdates loom largely. But it also gave us a tacit agreement of understanding. So now, when we get together, it's usually for a walk on the beach or a workout at Soul Cycle, with a limit on our after-activity alcohol consumption.

What really happened was that we all become a little more proactive in our quest for healthier and happier lives. There doesn't seem to be a reason in the world to accept that heart disease, high blood pressure, high cholesterol, diabetes, obesity, and cancer are inevitable. What we have reason to believe is that, through education and positive health choices, we can alter our lives. A confident V is a standard by which we can measure the health of our bodies and minds. A confident V is our ideal role model. Care for your V and you will care for and about yourself as a whole woman. I promise.

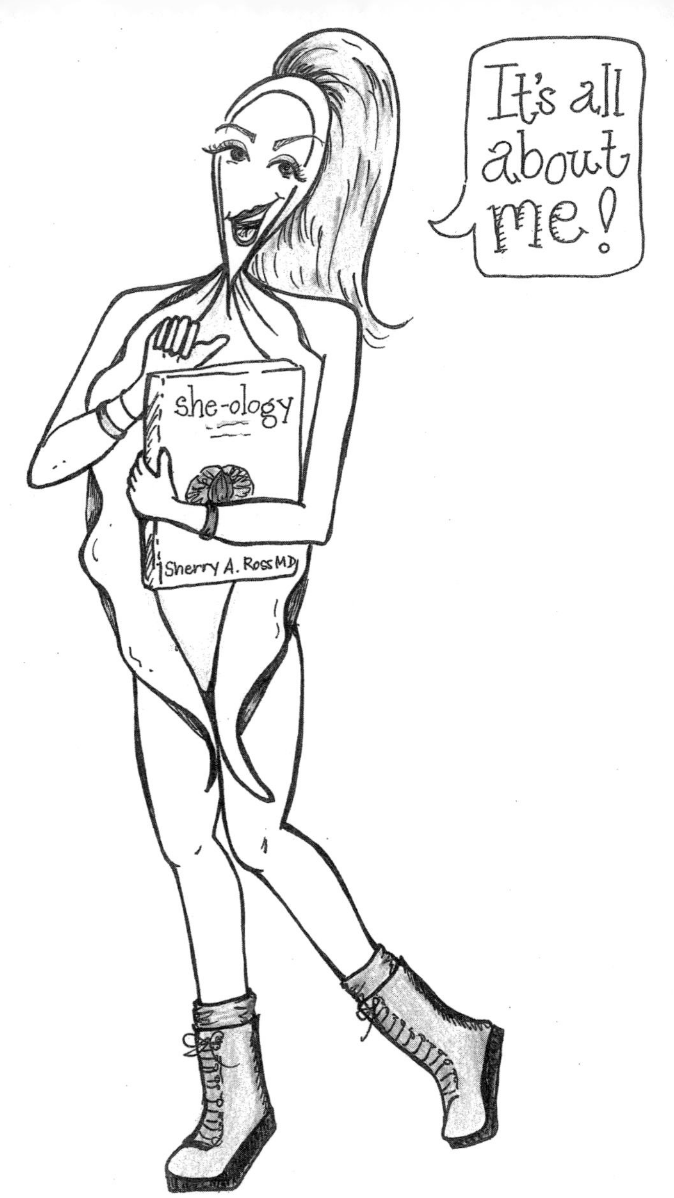

It's all about me!
she-ology
Sherry A. Ross MD

CHAPTER 2

# take charge

"My mother passed away when I was a young girl and my father never remarried, so I went through my adolescence having no older woman I could talk to about my body, its needs, and my sexual health. Left to my own devices, I scoured the internet, landing on heaps of misinformation.

When I was fourteen, I developed a yeast infection from taking antibiotics. I read on a website that if I put yogurt up my vagina, I'd be cured. So I slathered on a Greek variant—after soaking in a warm bath—both of which actually made the infection much worse. In fact, I ended up in an emergency room because of the pain.

Afterward, I realized not only were conversations about vaginal health lacking in Sex Ed classes, but there was a general societal shame in talking about anything vagina-related. I had friends that suffered through bladder infections because they were too embarrassed to seek help or talk to a parent.

There are billions of vaginas on this planet, which makes me wonder why we have such a difficult time talking about them, especially since it's through them that new life is brought into this world.

Because of that, I urge you to be a proud vagina owner. Give your vagina the love and respect and care that you reserve for the most cherished things in your life. Realize the potentially dangerous consequences of disregarding your vagina and your body as a whole.

How might you begin? Well, if you're sexually active, start with STI screenings *every six months*. I tend to get tested with every new partner, but I realize this may not be a financially viable option for everyone. However, in most cities there are free testing clinics. Planned Parenthood does a great job of working with you and making care affordable. Even if you are in a monogamous relationship, you should get tested regularly. It only takes one presumably innocent slip-up on your partner's end to threaten your health. Your safety comes first. I also strongly push for condom use unless you are in a mutually monogamous, tested relationship.

If you don't plan on becoming pregnant, you're in luck because, these days, women have various birth control options. In fact, I'm on my third Skyla-brand IUD. Before that, I used the NuvaRing and birth control pills. Taking control of my own method of birth control alleviates the worry of pregnancy, enabling me to be more present in my sexual experiences!

So that's all for me right now because Dr. Sherry will take it from here. She is a go-to source of information I wish I'd had when I started searching for answers about my vagina and my own sexuality. The fact is that vaginas are amazing!”

—**Eileen Kelly** Millennial Sex Expert

## Take Charge V

In her must-read essay, "The female price of male pleasure," Lili Loofbourow responds to the question as to why a woman wouldn't get out of an uncomfortable sexual situation as soon as she felt discomfort. Loofbourow answers: "Women are enculturated to be uncomfortable most of the time. And to ignore their discomfort... [To quote] David Foster Wallace: 'This is the water we swim in.'"

This water, this atmosphere, this culture in which women have historically taken a back seat, has never been more apparent than when it comes to a woman's needs. Obviously, that back seat has not been *chosen* by women; rather, it has been the only seat offered to women for centuries, especially when it has come to women's biological, medical, and sexual needs.

The messages that women get about sex and about embracing their own sexuality without judgment, embarrassment, or shame are confusing, at best, and dangerous, at worst. Sexual education is not just about learning about birth control and the names of body parts; it's about pride and pleasure and empowerment. Women have been taught for too long a time that their sexual needs are not important, that they're not the priority in a relationship, and that they're certainly not the main event in the bedroom. You have it heard before: "Sex is for men" or "Men need sex more than women." There is a social inequality under the sheets that we need to acknowledge and redefine. It's our right to be sexually satisfied and proud of it.

Unfortunately, as important as women's sexual health is, it is not often put at the top of a woman's "to do" list. Between the stress of kids, work, career, finances, and generally keeping a dozen or so balls in the air at a time, women are not paying the attention to their own sexual health that they need to.

Not only are women not making their sexual health a priority, they're not *talking* about their sexual health and concerns, not even with their closest girlfriends—even though statistics show that four out of ten of those girlfriends are having some sexual concerns and difficulties, and 10 to 20 percent of them have never had an orgasm.

If you're hesitant to talk about sex and sexual dysfunction with your partner or your BFF, you're probably equally hesitant (if not more so) to talk about it with your health care provider. But that's where the conversation ought to begin!

*At nineteen, Sophie came to see me for her first gynecological exam. She seemed quite comfortable sitting across from me in my office asking pointed questions that she'd come up with in advance of our appointment. She told me that she had been with her one and only boyfriend, Scottie, for two years, and that neither had been sexually active before their relationship. One question led to another, and it became clear that they fell into the same routine when it came to sex. They would kiss for less than a minute, then Scottie would touch her breasts, and then, every once in a while, he would gently touch her clitoris. Apparently, Scottie always had an erection before the kissing even started and could only last about five minutes before "shooting his wad." Needless to say, Sophie never had an orgasm with Scottie. She needed to know if there was something wrong with her.*

## On Your Mark, Get Ready, Set...*Come*

Here are the facts: On average, it takes men five minutes to achieve orgasm. Not surprisingly, it takes a whole twenty minutes for women to do the same. *This* is where foreplay becomes the key ingredient to success.

Sophie's Scottie, like so many other *bros*, had no clue as to those statistics. I told Sophie that it was up to her to educate Scottie if he cared about pleasing her in bed—and, if he didn't want to please her, well, then, something in the relationship was amiss.

Sophie is actually in the norm when it comes to an inability to orgasm with vaginal intercourse. Roughly, only 25 percent of women can have an orgasm during vaginal intercourse alone. The other 75 percent need some sort of clitoral stimulation to have an orgasm.

Maybe it's time to try something new. Maybe you ought to experiment with being on top during vaginal intercourse so that your partner can stimulate your clitoris with his hand during penetration, because clitoral stimulation is key, whether by caressing or licking. A lubricant such as extra virgin coconut oil or olive oil can heighten the pleasure of touch and even help bring on an orgasm more quickly. If, after such stimulation, orgasm is still not in the making, there may be inhibiting factors involved.

The following can inhibit orgasm:

* Alcohol
* Certain medications, including antidepressants, anti-anxiety, narcotics, and mood-altering drugs
* Fatigue
* Stress
* Depression, anxiety, or other emotional speed bumps
* Sexual inhibition

All of this points to why communication with your partner is vital.

Look, the truth is that all of us are a product of our upbringing—our parents, siblings, best friends, partners past and present, and, for some of us, our religion. Oftentimes, what's forgotten in that upbringing is the encouragement to explore sexuality. I find this ironic since *sexuality* is as part of our lives as eating and sleeping.

You must understand your own sexuality and know what feels good to you before you can help your partner to understand. I am a huge fan of using masturbation as exploration, so you can learn how to have an orgasm on your own *before* expecting your partner to provide you with one.

Culturally, women are meant to just go with the flow when it comes to sex, but that has become an archaic ideal. There's no better time than now to take charge in the bedroom and with your own sexual health. Discomfort with penetration sex is *not* typical, and, if your partner can't give you an orgasm, it is significant and warrants work on *his* part. "Faking it" just to please your partner is *out,* and the acknowledgment of your own feelings and needs in a healthy sexual relationship is *in.*

It's true women and men are wired differently, especially in their sexuality. Psychologist Roy Baumeister, an expert in sexual health and gender differences, believes that men have a stronger sex drive. He explains, "Men are different, which doesn't mean they don't crave intimacy, love, and connection. Their sex drive is just more straightforward—for them the connections come from *having* sex."

Therein lies a lot of the disconnect for men. Even if their sex drive is more straightforward, at the very least, they must understand what women want and need before getting naked with them. A man has to learn about his partner's sexual behavior—and that behavior is different in every woman. It's not like one behavior or size fits all, as is the message men have been given by the onslaught of pornography.

Men, listen up: The women in porn do not mirror the women in real life. Porn is not a reference for what women want in bed. In fact, porn only supports all the misconceptions there are about sex and messes with our romantic and sexual relationships. As Dr. Gail Dines, a professor of sociology and a modern-day hero and leading anti-porn feminist says, "Porn sites get more visitors than Netflix, Amazon, and Twitter combined each month. We basically need to bring down the 'porn monster' that has taught our girls and boys what is wrong in the bedroom."

Speaking of our boys and girls, I bought all three of my sons the book, *She Comes First: The Thinking Man's Guide to Pleasuring a Woman* by Ian Kerner, when they were teenagers. Yes, for sure, they were silently mortified when I gave each their own copy—separately, at least—but I felt it was my responsibility to help enlighten their paths in the bedroom, so to speak.

> *"For women, the best aphrodisiacs are words. The G-spot is in the ears. He who looks for it below there is wasting his time."*
>
> —Isabel Allende, *Of Love and Shadows*

What's important is that *you* know what feels good and what doesn't. Intimacy and sexual satisfaction are basic, instinctual human needs. You must help your partner by verbalizing what feels good, but, in order to do that, you must be able to say it to yourself.

## Empowering Young Women

The topic of sex education in the classroom has been, and remains today, a controversial subject, the parameters of which depend on the state where you live and the philosophy of your local school district. Although it's proven that sex education, if taught properly, can reduce risky sexual behavior and experiences, there are states and school districts that refuse to believe so.

This must change. It doesn't take a PhD to explain the ins and outs of Sex Ed. It doesn't matter whether a Sex Ed teacher is the school's biology teacher or the gym instructor, as long as they have had the proper training to give out accurate and age-appropriate sexual health information.

Imagine if there was an informed teacher who could say to your daughters (and sons): What questions should you ask yourself before having sex for the first time? How great would it be for a young person to be able to ask herself the following?

* Are you ready to have sex with this person?
* Is it consensual?
* Have you talked about safe sex and the importance of using a condom?
* Are you on birth control?
* Are you in an emotionally and physically healthy relationship?

This is an example of the type of education needed in our children's schools, for the sake of your daughters and for your sons.

## Taking Matters Into Your Own Hands

*Harper, a conscientious sixteen-year-old high school junior, came to see me for her first gynecological exam. She was a self-described nerd who was always at the top of her class and had her sights set on an Ivy League college. Part of the reason why she came to see me was because she was worried. She thought about sex all the time and loved to masturbate, so she needed to ask someone in the know: "Am I a sex fiend?"*

I asked Harper if her affinity for masturbation affected her ability to be successful in school or whether it affected her daily routine. She said it didn't and, in fact, it made her feel good about herself and helped her to sleep like a baby at night. I told Harper that I was really proud of her for learning about her body and embracing her sexual health.

After all, masturbation is the best way to understand your own body and to find out what brings you pleasure. Not only is it a completely normal part of adolescence, it is also usually the first sexual experience a person will have. By literally taking matters into your own hands, you can be on your way towards getting in touch with what pleases you sexually, no matter your age. By learning what gives you pleasure, you can provide your partner with a successful roadmap in bed because, let's face it, you cannot expect your partner to find what gives you sexual pleasure if you don't know it yourself.

Still need convincing? Masturbation not only makes you feel good...

* It is a normal and healthy sexual activity that's pleasurable and safe.

* It's a perfect way to release sexual tension and stress.
* It improves sexual health and relationships.
* It's a natural sleeping pill.
* It's a guaranteed way to avoid getting a sexually transmitted infection or pregnant.

As much as I believe that a woman must learn early on—by her late teens, early twenties—about her body and what makes her feel good, I also believe that it's never too late for any woman to educate herself about her erogenous zones.

## Secrets to an Orgasm, or, Penis Need Not Apply

Foreplay! Foreplay! Foreplay...and more foreplay!

Romancing the clitoris is commandment number one in achieving orgasm. In order to do that, you must get to know and understand the clitoris—with its 8,000 nerve fibers—whose one and only job is to provide a woman with sexual pleasure, better known as The Big O!

We already know the way to sexually arousing a woman is to appeal to her "other" sex organ, the one *above* her shoulders—her mind—so it shouldn't come as a surprise that most women want and need more time to build up to arousal. How much time, you ask? Research has it that the average foreplay in the United States lasts about thirteen minutes, but research by the definitive human sexual response pioneers Masters and Johnson shows that it ought to last eighteen or nineteen minutes (at least). Something, somewhere is falling *short*.

I love what Dr. Lindsey Doe, Host of YouTube's *Sexplanations,* says about foreplay: "Foreplay doesn't have to build up to something more important. It can *be* what's more important. Most of us probably think of kissing or touching our partner's genitals when we're thinking foreplay. But it's 2017—use your imagination."

So where does the breakdown in bed happen? Why are women not getting enough foreplay with their partners? Perhaps we don't leave enough time for sex. Think about it: How can we slow down in the bedroom when most of us have a problem slowing down in all other aspects of life? Twenty minutes for foreplay plus orgasm might not seem like much time, but, in fact, it can seem like an eternity in the course of an already-hectic, time-deprived day.

Dr. Emily Nagoski, award-winning author of the New York Times bestseller, *Come As You Are: The Surprising New Science That Will Transform Your Sex Life* goes deep into the discussion of foreplay. She writes, "We're taught, from the very beginning in our culture, a model of sexual response that is based entirely on how men work, and so [the assumption goes] the extent to which women fail to be like men is the extent to which they fail to be sexually normal, and that's just not true.... The standards, for me, for healthy, normal sex are consent, lack of unwanted pain and satisfaction. When all three of those things are there, you're doing really well. Satisfaction's complicated, though, because that's based on, 'I have an expectation of what it should be like and I either do or don't match that expectation.' And if your expectations are based on incorrect information, then you're going to be dissatisfied, not for medical reasons, but because your expectation doesn't make sense for who your body actually is."

## Exercise-Induced Orgasm

Among the many health benefits of exercising we can now be sure to add *orgasm*, since there is an undeniable connection between the strength of abdominal wall and pelvic floor muscles—which are strengthened with exercise as well as Kegels—and the ability to orgasm. Whether you are aware of it or not, by contracting and tightening your abdominal muscles you are also contracting and tightening your pelvic floor muscles, which can lead to what's known as a coregasm, an orgasm that happens while you're doing a core exercise or workout. In fact, up to 10 percent of women and men experience this type of orgasm while performing certain exercises.

Exercises involving the abdominal muscles—and are thereby most associated with coregasms—include weight lifting, yoga, spinning/bicycling, running, hiking, and walking. Some women can have coregasms while doing sit-ups, pull-ups, and chin-ups, or while climbing poles or ropes. What a perfect and healthy way of multitasking!

Beyond such types of exercising to achieve coregasm and to strengthen your pelvic floor muscles, there are even more intimate ways to educate yourself in the anatomy of arousal.

## Vaginal Mapping

I was recently asked to contribute to an international women's fashion magazine considered to be at the forefront of getting out the word on "Vaginal Mapping," which refers to a technique of receiving help in becoming familiar with your genitals in a way that is not only pleasant but *not* medical, clinical, sexual, or unexpected. It's a way of getting to intimately know your vagina, vulva, and pelvic floor.

## Take Charge V

The very existence of Vaginal Mapping shows how far women these days have come in their sexual awakening. In fact, women have described Vaginal Mapping—which not only utilizes touch, but mindfulness and breathing techniques—as a way of becoming truly relaxed, aware, and present in the moment.

Vaginal Mapping uses purpose and intention as a means of getting to know all parts that make you female. Breast mapping is also included in this vaginal awakening process. To me, this "mapping" process is simply code for learning to embrace your femininity and your sexual health without shame. It's all about getting to your know body from head to toe and experiencing a full body awakening.

Having a physical and emotional relationship with your vagina and learning about the ins and outs of your body and your sexuality at an early age will probably save you money on your therapy bills as an adult. However, instead of paying up to $1,200 for three sessions of vaginal mapping, why not learn about your own body for free?

I often pull out a mirror to my new teen patients while their legs are in stirrups in order to go over the vulvar area, so they know where a tampon goes, where urine comes out, and where the clitoris is. Everyone needs a roadmap, because understanding your vagina, clitoris, and your pelvis will help avoid problems relating to sexual dysfunction and disconnect with your own body.

I can't tell you the number of young women who have *never* looked at their anatomy, and the number of women who have been in sexual relationships yet have never masturbated or had an orgasm. It is imperative, at any age, to be aware of every part of your body without fear, inhibition, or embarrassment, and to know what makes your sexuality tick.

## Erogenous Zones: No Need to Yield!

There's no way to talk about sexuality without talking about the *erogenous zones,* which are basically any area of your body with a heightened sensitivity, so that, when stimulated, elicit a sexual response.

Your mouth, neck, ears, lips, nipples, back, hands, and lower stomach are typically areas of pleasure—erogenous zones. But there are other areas of the body that are also worth exploring, including ear lobes, hair, scalp, armpits, bottoms of feet, inner wrists, buttocks, and behind the knees. It may be a good idea to take notice of these oft-neglected zones as well.

In fact, why not make a date to be uninterrupted and naked with your partner for a day in order to explore all the nooks and crannies of each other's bodies? You can even mix it up in the bedroom by bringing some of your favorite "fun" foods—say, oldies but goodies such as whip cream, honey, caramel, or chocolate syrup. Take chances, explore, enjoy, and don't hold back on the pleasure of having your cake and eating it too!

## Sexual Activity and Virginity: Where is the Crossover?

When I was growing up, the term "virgin" referred to a person who had never had sexual intercourse—for girls, that meant having an intact hymen—but it also referred to one who was not engaged in *sexual activity.* In today's world, I think that the definition of a virgin seems to be outdated, at best.

Hearing that some of my teenage patients believed they were still *virgins,* even though they were having oral or anal sex, was the first thing that prompted me to reconsider the definition of virginity. Virginity certainly does not preclude sexual activity. What counts as sexual activity is the exchange of any kind of bodily fluid—including kissing! That exchange of fluids also happens when a penis enters the mouth, vagina, or rectum—all of which constitute sexual activity.

If you are part of the LGBT community, you may not *ever* have had sexual intercourse—especially since that term usually refers to sex between a man and a woman—but you may be sexually active. The definition of losing one's virginity is complicated and personal. It means different things to different people. It's really up to you to decide what losing your virginity means.

When you are ready to be sexually active with a person you feel comfortable and safe with, then it's the right time to engage in sexual activity. Don't ever let anyone make the decision for you as to when you should become sexually active. "Don't worry, you'll still be a virgin" is not a reason to let someone coerce you into a sexually active relationship that includes everything but sexual intercourse. Virginity is not the point. The point is to make the decision on your own, when you're ready.

## Protect Yourself Against Pregnancy

If you are ready to engage in sexual intercourse, and you do not want to become pregnant, luckily, there are many choices of birth control. It's a matter of finding the one that works best for you. To do that, I suggest making an appointment with your health care provider at least three months before having sex (if that is possible) to go over the different options.

Oral contraception, simply referred to as "the Pill," is still the most popular method of birth control in the United States. There are many different brands of OCPs (oral contraceptive pills), all of which combine different doses of the hormones estrogen and progesterone. The advantage to a pill is that, when you're ready to become pregnant, you can stop taking the pill on your own—although it's recommended that you wait a couple cycles before actively trying to become pregnant.

If you find that, for whatever reason, the pill is not for you, the IUD is a safe, effective and long-term contraception alternative. Even though the IUD has been around a long time, for many women it is the "new kid" on the block, since new, advanced technology has made it safer for women of all ages. Other long acting birth control methods available to women include Nexplanon, the arm implant, and the injectable Depo Provera, which last up to three years and must be removed if you plan on trying to become pregnant.

No matter what type of contraception you use, you're still responsible for taking matters into your own hands in protecting yourself against STIs (sexually transmitted infections).

## Protect Yourself Against Sexually Transmitted Infections

Before you start a sexual relationship, even if you and your partner "feel certain" that neither of you have any STIs, it's important for you both to be screened in order to *be certain*—remember, STIs may be asymptomatic or, as yet, undiagnosed. That out of the way, you still need to protect yourself, always, unless the two of you firmly commit to being monogamous.

Of course, the most effective way to protect against STIs is to abstain from any sexual activity, especially sexual intercourse, but that is neither the most practical nor the most enjoyable method of protection. However, insisting that your partner wear a condom at all times is the next best thing.

Condoms are the best way to help prevent sexually transmitted infections, pregnancy, HIV infections, and related diseases such as cervical cancer. No, it's not guaranteed to be 100 percent protection—if your partner has HPV or a herpes sore at the base of his penis and the condom slips off, you could be exposed to these viruses during sex—but, if you're sexually active, it *is* your best chance of preventing unwanted surprises. I feel strongly that you have to get into the habit of making a new partner wear a condom, at all times, until you make the decision to be completely monogamous. And remember to get your HPV vaccine in your tweens, in order to give you an added level of protection.

For same-sex partners, condoms are equally important, as are dental dams—which should be used during oral sex in order to protect the throat from HPV—since safe sex means condom use during vaginal or anal intercourse and oral sex. No excuses here—if there isn't a dental dam in grabbing distance, plastic wrap or a cut condom will do the trick.

Finally, no matter whether you've been with your partner one week or one year, safe sex practices remain the same. Your partner must wear a condom until they (and you) are 100 percent sure the relationship is completely monogamous. I don't want to be a cynic, but, even if an engagement ring is placed on the fourth finger of your left hand, make certain that gesture means complete monogamy.

## LGBTQI and Sex Education

Sadly, sex education in high school tends to be geared only toward straight, cisgender teens. In fact, a 2015 survey of millennials reported that only 12 percent said their sex education classes covered same-sex relationships. Teens that fall into the LGBTQI category have to look beyond the walls of high school for accurate and reliable information related to their *sexual preferences*. Research also shows that LGBTQ youth have a limited number of trusted adults they feel comfortable talking with about *sexual health*, which means they have to find reliable information online or from peers.

With sexual fluidity more prominent in today's youth culture, there needs to be greater access to reliable information on alternative sexual lifestyles. Such information is critical in understanding one's personal needs and the parameters of healthy sexual experiences. One such source is the local Gay and Lesbian Center—most major cities have at least one such center—where teens (and parents) may find resources for LGBTQ high school students. Other organizations such as Advocates for Youth, Answer, GLSEN (Gay, Lesbian and Straight Education Network), the Human Rights Campaign, Planned Parenthood Federation of America, and the Sexuality Information and Education Council of the US (SIECUS) can help provide LGBT students with information on sex education or, at least, direct them to reliable resources.

Sexuality is an important aspect of our well-being, and as important in a healthy romantic relationship as love and affection. We seldom think of sex as something that *isn't* instinctual, but the fact is that enjoyable sex is learned. Sure, instinct is involved somewhat, as is a dusting of magic, but one doesn't magically have an orgasm without taking an active role. Before you can have a healthy relationship with another person, you have to have a healthy relationship with yourself.

Young women need to empower themselves to help make a cultural shift in sexual societal norms. They must rewrite the traditional "rules" that have, for so long, neglected the sexual needs of women, be they straight, gay, trans, or cis. Women, take control; take *authorship*.

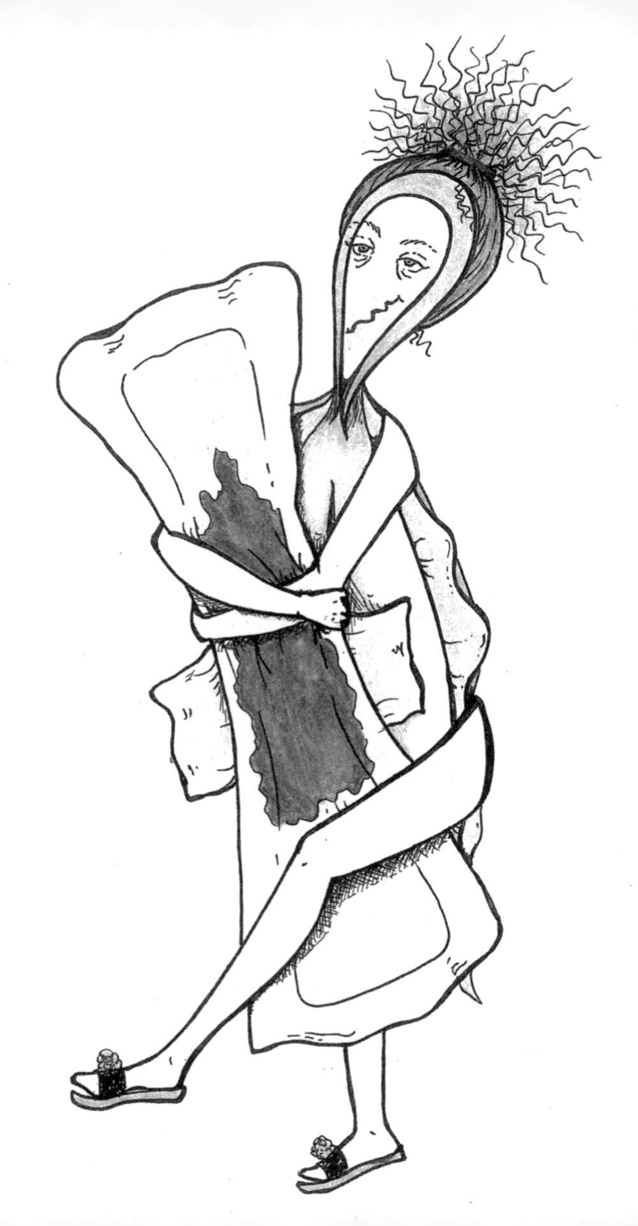

## CHAPTER 3

# bloody

"I'd been having one of *those* conversations—you know, the one where you compare notes with a good girlfriend about the intense period pain and cramping and heavy bleeding that you've kinda had your whole life, but didn't deal with because there were just too many more *important* things to take care of? But, by then, the pain of those crazy periods had become so bad that I could barely leave the house on certain days of the month. Fortunately for me, the particular girlfriend I was talking to happened to be a longtime patient of Dr. Sherry's, and she insisted I see her 'amazing' doctor that I was 'sure to love.' Okay, I thought. I had nothing to lose, except maybe for the pain.

During one of my first appointments with Dr. Sherry, she found two big fibroids on my uterus. I'd suffered from fibroids twenty years earlier, but I had surgery to remove them. What I hadn't known then was that, with fibroids, there's always a chance they'll come back. Twenty years and three tests later, they did.

A little backstory: Because fibroids grow (and shrink) with estrogen production, they didn't give me any trouble during my three pregnancies. Instead, they were kind of hiding, in wait, but, when they returned, they returned with a vengeance, which brings me back to Dr. Sherry.

When Dr. Sherry found those fibroids, instead of sending me off to have surgery (which was fairly standard practice twenty years earlier) she talked me through all my options—of which there were many. Because she was up on all the advances in gynecological care, she helped me weigh all those options. Nowadays, fibroids can be embolized—a minimally invasive procedure that helps shrink them—removed laparoscopically or robotically, or treated with medication. With these procedures comes a quicker recovery time—which is important for me, because I have three kids to run after, along with a fairly chock-full career.

What I ultimately learned was that I could no longer put my head in the sand and avoid my own health care. It's Dr. Sherry who never ceases to remind me that I have to put on my own oxygen mask before I can help others. She has put me at ease in talking about any and all of my health concerns, especially those potentially embarrassing ones. And who doesn't need a doctor like that?”

—**Holly Coombs** Actress, TV Producer

## Period Parties Add This…

Just the facts on our monthly bloody valentines: A healthy woman under the age of fifty-one that does not suffer from any medical conditions or hormonal imbalances, such as perimenopause, or is not taking any medications—because medications *can* interfere with the menstrual cycle—ought to be getting a period every twenty-one to thirty-five days. In fact, that twenty-one-to-thirty-five-day window is true for 80 percent of women. As far as the *duration* is concerned, most women with regular menstrual cycles can expect a period lasting three to five days, but one woman's *normal* may be as few as one day or as many as seven.

For many women, *normal* also means an increase of irritability and anxiety right before periods. Add to that increase of emotional instability a late period, spotting mid-cycle, and an increased flow or frequency, there's no wonder for the occasional *freak out* around our often-mystifying menstrual cycles. So, firstly, I'd like to try to de-mystify the whole process of menstruation, starting with puberty.

## Puberty: The Introduction to Our Normal Hormonal Cycles

For women, puberty usually begins around the age of eight, when the pituitary gland sends signals to the ovaries to produce the hormones estrogen and progesterone—the two main hormones of the female reproductive system and, in fact, the most important hormones in the development and maintenance of female organs and characteristics.

The first sign of puberty is the development of breast buds—due to the start of estrogen stimulating breast tissue—which is accompanied by the appearance of hair under the arms and on the legs and vagina, and, unfortunately, facial acne. Six months prior to a girl's first period she will probably notice a clear vaginal discharge, then, at around eleven or twelve, she may experience her first cycle and it's *Hello, Flo*!

### *The Cycle*

A menstrual cycle consists of four distinct phases: menstruation, the follicular phase, ovulation, and the luteal phase.

During the follicular phase, the follicles in the ovary mature, leading to ovulation. Ovulation occurs around Day Fourteen, at which time an ovarian follicle has produced an egg, which can then be fertilized by sperm. This is the time when pregnancy may occur, although the egg is available to be fertilized for only twenty-four hours before it disintegrates. The luteal phase then begins, during which estrogen and progesterone increase and thicken the lining of the uterus to prepare it to accept an embryo. If an egg hasn't been fertilized, it means that a pregnancy has not taken place. When a pregnancy doesn't happen, estrogen and progesterone levels drop, and the thickened lining of the uterus—which would have supported a pregnancy—is no longer needed, so it sheds through the vagina in what we know as the menstrual period, thereby marking an end to the luteal phase.

During your period, you experience the release of the combination of blood, mucous, and tissue from the uterus. It's also during your period when you are most likely to suffer the *normal symptoms* of cramps, lower abdominal or back pain, bloating, tender breasts, mood swings, food cravings, and headaches. Many women also experience gas and diarrhea a couple days before and during their periods. Yes, it sounds like quite a party. As a side note: Many parents are now choosing to throw their daughters "period parties" in order to make the occasion of the onset of one's period celebratory rather than fearsome. In fact, many participants claim that those parties have provided them with powerful feelings of community and female strength. I say, don't knock it until you've tried—or attended—one! Which leads me to...

### *The Conversation*

Of course, I'm referring to the conversation that a mother (or father, in some instances) has with her or his daughter about puberty and menstruation—a sensitive subject, if ever there was one. It can be rough and awkward going all around, I know, which is why it's important to try to develop a way to ease your daughter into talking about her body and the changes associated with puberty *before* her first period. In regard to this, preparation is your best weapon.

### *The Puberty Prep*

* Like the Scouting motto—*be prepared!* You need to know the signs and symptoms of puberty so that you can best prepare your daughter for what's to come. Don't get caught like a deer in the headlights when she comes to you with her first questions!
* Have the conversation. Since breast buds are usually the first sign of puberty, the appearance of them—around age eight—is a good time to start the conversation about what to expect with puberty. Begin by letting your daughter know that the changes she'll start to see are perfectly normal, beginning with those breast buds—small bumps in the breast area, similar in size to peanut M & M's—which are the beginning of breast tissue. Let her know that these bumps can feel tender as the tissue continues to grow. Talk to her about buying a training bra, which will help support the growing tissue, and may also help to make her feel more comfortable (or

less self-conscious) than she might in an undershirt. Mention how she'll start to see the development of hair under her arms and on her legs and vagina. And, while you're at it, this is a great opportunity to discuss some good hygiene habits. Talk about keeping those areas clean with mild soap and water.

* Let your daughter know that you're available to answer all her questions and address any concerns she may have. You may or may not want to launch into a full, detailed conversation about her period at this same time, as it could be too much information for one sitting, but don't wait too long to circle back to it as she may wind up getting all her information (rightly or wrongly) from the internet.
* Speaking of internet information, the one thing that your daughter will not glean from a Google search (unless you're an over-sharing Mommy Blogger) is your own, personal experience of puberty and menstruation. Ease her anxiety by sharing your own observations and the trepidation you may have had about your own changing body, and what you learned during the process. Ask how she's feeling about getting her period. If she's not quite ready to talk, or she's disinterested in the topic, or she's just plain embarrassed, try back in a few weeks or months. At least open the door to discussion. Let her know you're there when she's ready to talk.
* Aside from your own hard-earned wisdom and experience, don't be afraid to employ some age-appropriate books and videos on the subject of puberty and female anatomy. Your daughter may not seem ready to talk,

but she may be ready to take a look at a good, instructive book geared towards her particular age group. She may then come to you for some edification and wide-eyed questioning.

* Lastly, be sure to promote body confidence, not fear. Teach your daughter about her body, and please, please use the correct terms when talking about her breasts, vagina, period, et al. Sure, you may encounter some giggles and eye rolls—that's completely normal—but it's important for women of all ages to be able to properly (and confidently) identify their female anatomy. It's something you'll need to do for the rest of your life.

We need to normalize the conversation about female anatomy and physiology. Start by talking to your daughter and setting a positive example of what that conversation might be. We owe it to our daughters and ourselves.

## Period Abnormalities

As with any bodily function, abnormalities in periods can crop up, and sometimes it's difficult to tell whether that abnormality is a *red flag* for a condition that may be temporary or chronic, serious or otherwise.

### *Common Red Flags*

*Lori Jean, a forty-something patient with a fourteen-year-old daughter, is an artist who specializes in giant, over-sized sculptures—which means that she has had to have the strength, both mentally and, especially, physically, to succeed in her personal and professional life. So, when Lori Jean came to me with complaints of an irregular period accompanied by fatigue and impatience with her daughter, she wasn't sure if the problem was with her or her daughter's raging teen hormones. She also mentioned trouble sleeping and bouts of feeling particularly hot and sweaty, and her periods were coming every two weeks and lasting seven to ten days. Her previous doctor dismissed the symptoms as "normal for a woman in her forties." No whys or wherefores! When she came to me for a second opinion, I checked her FSH and Estradiol levels, which confirmed that she was in perimenopause. She was not "The World's Worst Mom," as she'd formerly concluded! In fact, once her "condition" was diagnosed, help was readily available.*

Lori Jean's story is important in realizing that most every "abnormality" in your usual physical and emotional self is not only diagnosable, it can be availed with treatment. For Lori Jean, that meant a low-dose birth control pill. The point is that you know your body better than anyone, so, when you feel out of sorts, it's best to consult with your health care provider in order to find out the reason for your concerns or discomfort.

With regard to period abnormalities, red flags may be subtle or monumental. You may be concerned because your period is suddenly irregular, or lasts much longer than usual, or the blood flow is noticeably diminished or heavier—heavy bleeding would be characterized by large blood clots the size of grapes, or a flow that requires pad or tampon changes every thirty to sixty minutes over the course of a few hours. Perhaps the severity of your PMS symptoms has increased and cramps are starting to cramp your daily style. Is brown spotting continuing over the course of a few months? Maybe you've noticed mood swings or the onset of migraines. Whether you're fifteen or fifty, if any of these symptoms are enough to cause you to miss school, work, workouts, or social engagements, or make you confused or frustrated, it's time to check out the possible causes—and I don't mean with Dr. Google—because there are myriad common causes of irregular and heavy periods. These causes include:

* **Thyroid Dysfunction**
* **Polycystic Ovarian Syndrome (PCOS):** A hormonal disorder, which may result in infrequent or prolonged periods.
* **Perimenopause:** Refers to the years in the reproductive life cycle, during which ovarian function becomes irregular and periods become erratic (and frustrating!). This hormonal cycle usually occurs between the ages of forty and fifty-five and is the precursor to menopause.
* **Menopause:** This natural hormonal cycle occurs when the ovaries stop producing estrogen and female hormones are completely depleted. Once you stop having your period for a year, you are officially in menopause! Physical, hormonal, and psychological changes can be so disruptive as to involve medical intervention, so best to a checkup ASAP.
* **Uterine polyps and fibroids:** Uterine fibroids are the most common benign pelvic tumors in women. Also known as leiomyomas and myomas, the size, shape, and location of these muscle tumors can be found anywhere in and around the uterus and are typically seen in women aged thirty to forty. Common signs and symptoms include irregular and heavy bleeding, cramping, pelvic pain, and pressure during periods.

Uterine polyps are growths (usually benign) inside the uterine cavity that also cause irregular and heavy bleeding. A pelvic ultrasound is used to diagnosis these uterine abnormalities.

* **Excessive Exercising and Sudden Weight Changes:** Both these conditions can offset your hormone levels causing irregular periods. In particular, the hormone Leptin is produced in fatty tissue, so, with a drastic decrease in body fat, this (and other) hormones may *drop*, contributing to irregular periods. Extreme weight gain may *increase* estrogen levels, causing heavy periods and blood clots.
* **Physical or Emotional Stress:** Certainly not a surprise, significant stress—such as divorce or death of a loved one—can disrupt one's hormonal balance, creating delayed, irregular, or heavy periods.
* **Illness:** Medications used in treating a variety of illnesses may also cause a disruption of hormones. Thyroid medication, steroids, and antipsychotics, in particular, are a likely cause for period irregularities.
* **Pregnancy:** This hormonal cycle can be completely joyous or a disaster, depending on your planning or lack thereof.
* **Sexually Transmitted Infections (STIs)**
* **Excessive Alcohol Use:** Excessive alcohol use can increase levels of estrogen, disrupting hormones enough so as to cause irregular periods.

### *Period Interrupted—Amenorrhea*

*Not* having a period is *not* how our bodies are meant to function, from a hormonal perspective, so, if you haven't had a period by the time you reach seventeen, you may be facing a potential period problem.

Having a monthly a period suggests your body is in sync with itself and that your hormones are balanced. The older you get, the more magical this balance may seem, as regular periods can help to make you feel more emotionally and physically stable—and who can argue with that?

If you happen to go three or four months without a period, especially after experiencing regular periods, you are experiencing amenorrhea. Unless you were planning on getting pregnant, amenorrhea can definitely be one of those red flags we talked about.

The causes of Amenorrhea are many and varied, including:

* Pregnancy
* Breast feeding
* Thyroid disorder
* Polycystic Ovary Syndrome (PCOS)
* Perimenopause and menopause
* Continuous oral contraceptive use
* Progesterone birth control—including IUDs and Depo-Provera, Arm Implant (Nexplanon)
* Medication—including chemotherapy and psychotropic
* Excessive weight loss or weight gain
* Anorexia/Bulimia
* Malnutrition
* Excessive exercise
* Pituitary disorder and tumors
* Uterine adhesions
* Premature ovarian failure

* Radiation treatment
* Recreational drug abuse
* Depression and other psychiatric disorders
* Genetic disorders—including Turner Syndrome and Fragile X
* Excessive stress and anxiety
* Cushing Disease
* Congenital Adrenal Hyperplasia

When amenorrhea lasts three to four months (or longer), it's important to visit your health care provider for a general workup. Aside from a physical exam, she will ask for a detailed history of your physical and emotional changes as a means of finding the possible cause of your amenorrhea and what particular tests to order. Depending upon the *cause*, treatment can then be determined.

Regaining a regular period may often simply involve hormones, such as the birth control pill or progesterone, but some women have had success with acupressure and homeopathic alternatives. Again, speak with your health care provider to discuss your options.

### *Birth Control and No Period*

Of all the possible side effects of the birth control pill, the most welcome is light or non-existent periods. Progesterone IUDs, such as the brands Mirena, Kyleena, Skyla, and Liletta may also make your period light or non-existent. These are expected side effects that are especially welcome for women with heavy or irregular periods.

However, when some women *stop* taking the Pill, their periods may take one to three months to return to normal.

Since many young women start the Pill in their teens—before they have a good idea of the *regularity* of their periods—they won't know what is regular or suspect in their period cycles when they go off the Pill. Going off the Pill does not in itself *cause* amenorrhea. If you go off the Pill and then don't have a period, that is not normal. In fact, you may have an underlying hormonal problem that has been masked by taking the birth control pill.

Normal period bleeding should happen at regular time intervals as a result of naturally occurring hormonal changes in our bodies. These hormonal changes make our periods come at predictable times of the month.

If your period does not come at these predicted times, this may suggest there is an underlying problem with your hormones and seeing a health care provider would be recommended. Whatever you do, please don't rely on folklore or myth when it comes to period realities. That said, here are some of those myths:

### *Common Period Myths*

* **Missing a period is a sure sign of illness or disease.** *Whoa, Nelly.* Don't panic. You could be pregnant or entering peri-menopause or menopause or the missed period is a side effect of birth control.
* **Having periods in sync with girlfriends in close proximity is an old wives' tale.** As an OB-GYN, I hear about sisters, mothers, and roommates getting their periods together all the time. Because I hear it so often, I *do* believe menstrual synchrony exists. In fact, the first study on menstrual synchrony, published in 1971, claims that it does exist. It showed that, when

women spend more than three months together, their periods start within four days of each other's. However, this study has not been duplicated through *controlled medical conditions* to support menstrual synchrony as a real phenomenon. But the fact is that, in my twenty-five years as a physician, I have learned that not everything that happens to us *medically* can be *proven* through scientific research. Case in point: When I was in college and living in the Delta Gamma Sorority house, my four roommates and I—soon after we began to live together—got our periods at the same time of the month. Go figure!

* **Plan B has nothing to do with my period.** Plan B—known as the "morning after pill"—is a form of emergency contraception after an "accident." By *accident*, I, of course, mean the lack of reliable birth control during sex. If you've had sex without protection and need a serious tactic to be certain of preventing pregnancy, the morning after pill can be used up to seventy-two hours after having sex—however, it is proven to be *89 percent effective* when taken within *twenty-four hours* of having sex. So, if Plan B is the way you must go, you may experience irregular spotting or bleeding lasting days or even weeks. It may take one or two months for your period to reset and go back to normal. Plan B can be a godsend, but a "Plan A"—contraception to avoid pregnancy in the first place—is a helluva lot less stressful!
* **Having sex can bring on your period early.** Spotting or bleeding after sex is common, but it does not always come from the vagina. It may be coming from the

cervix or urinary tract. If your full period does come early, after sex, it is most likely a result of coincidence or environmental or hormonal causes. Other causes may include sexually transmitted infection, trauma to the cervix or vagina, cervical polyp, pregnancy, or cervical infection, but, more than likely, some spotting or bleeding is not a great cause for concern.

It's so easy to jump to the worse-case scenario when it comes to *signs from the vagina,* but, before making yourself crazy, please consult with a health care provider. Meanwhile, do what you can to stay healthy and hormonally regulated.

Healthy lifestyle habits and rituals that can help include:

* Eating healthy foods, including fresh fruits and veggies, proteins such as fish and chicken, and complex carbohydrates such as whole grains and brown rice.
* Exercise! Exercise is often helpful for PMS symptoms and menstrual cramps, and the increase in "feel good," mood-boosting endorphins and serotonin during exercise help ease pain and stress any time of the month. Walking, jogging, Pilates, yoga, swimming... pick your passion.
* Green tea, a great natural diuretic as well as a comforting beverage for bloating, before, after, and during your period...or anytime, for that matter.
* Calcium-rich foods and supplements, which help reduce muscle cramping. The ideal amount of 1,000mg/day of calcium can be obtained with dairy products (cheese, yogurt, and milk), sunflower seeds, spinach, soybeans, kale, figs, almonds, sesame seeds, and tofu, all of which are excellent sources of calcium.

* Drinking water. This is a must for anyone, but did you know that drinking warm or hot water helps relax the uterine muscles?
* Aside from calcium, vitamins E, D, thiamine, magnesium, and omega 3-fish oil are helpful in relieving period bloat and swelling.
* Getting a good night sleep! Sleep is critical to good health—mentally and physically—especially in the couple weeks before your period. It is shown that most adults need seven to eight hours of sleep a night. Some people thrive on more, some on less, so it's up to you to determine what is best for you. No matter your need, *sleep deprivation* can affect your ability to be efficient in all aspects of your life. Everything from focus to reaction times, to clear thinking is compromised by a lack of sleep. Sleep deprivation can leave you emotionally raw, frustrated, moody, irritable, and stressed out, especially if you are already feeling hormonally challenged.
* Physical hygiene. Don't forget to clean your vulva and vagina every day with a non-fragrant, vagina-friendly soap. Remember that the use of tampons and sanitary pads can bring unwanted bacteria to this very sensitive and delicate area. The perfect daily soap for the delicate vulva and vagina is Summer's Eve Blissful Cleaning wash. What I like about Summer's Eve is that their products are clinically tested by gynecologists and dermatologists to make sure they are safe and hypoallergenic. They also have convenient cleansing cloths that can be used on-the-go, especially on those days when you can't shower after a workout or before being intimate with your partner, or when you're using

tampons or sanitary pads. In fact, as an alternative to those tampons and pads, why not try using a menstrual cup to collect blood during a period? Not only can they be left inside the vagina overnight and up to twelve hours, menstrual cups are a reusable, convenient, environmentally friendly, hypo-allergenic, less costly and healthy alternative to tampons and pads. My favorite is the Lunette Menstrual Cup, which is FDA-cleared, medical- grade extra-soft, with a number one safety rating with the Danish Consumer Counsel. Whether you use tampons, pads, or menstrual cups, change them regularly—especially tampons!

* Avoiding or limiting certain foods around your period time that are known to cause bloat: beans, broccoli, Brussels sprouts, cabbage, and cauliflower. When in doubt as to what foods to avoid, rule of thumb points to "b" and "c" vegetables (i.e., **b**eans, **b**roccoli, **c**abbage, etc.). Other bloating culprits include rich and fatty foods, whole grains, apples, peaches, pears, lettuce, and onions.
* Limiting alcohol consumption, especially since alcoholic beverages make bloating symptoms worse.
* Avoiding foods high in sodium (salt, ladies!). Salt is a huge contributor to bloating and weight gain, which means that many salty, ethnic foods, such as Chinese and Thai, are, literally, off the table if you're experiencing bloating.

Your menstrual cycle is a terrific barometer of your overall health and wellness. You're never too young (or too old) to pay attention to the different phases of your cycle in order to become more aware of your physical, physiological, and emotional shifts. Like the moon, we have different monthly phases, phases that are marked by our menstrual cycles. So, maybe next time you're on your "dreaded period," instead, think of it (and your cycle as a whole) as a microcosm of the cycle of your life...and embrace the flow!

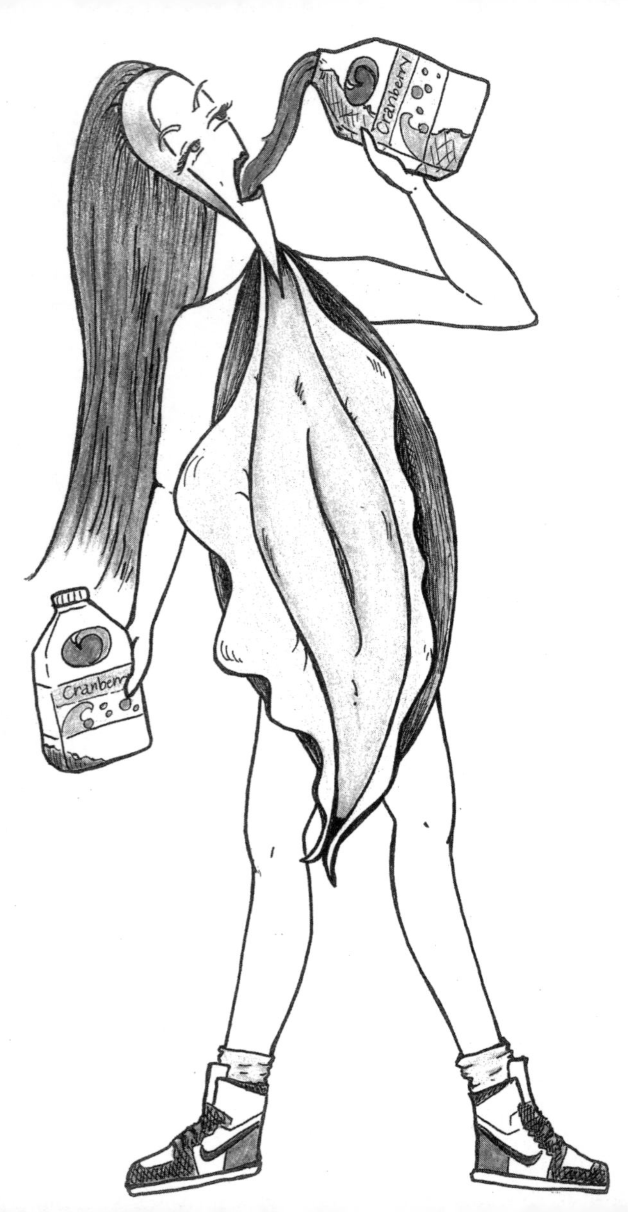

Cranberry
Cranberr

CHAPTER 4

# off tract

"Pregnancy was a shocker. I mean it was not the experience I was expecting. The hardest part for me was how my body became this whole other thing, and even though I was ecstatic about the life growing inside me, I felt physically horrible most of the time. Smells made me nauseous, even the smell of clean clothes! And my libido—no one told me that would disappear as quickly as did my waistline.

After my baby was born—and I had a parachute hanging where my flat tummy had once been—I felt bombarded with images in magazines and on social media reinforcing this myth of how my post-pregnancy body should apparently look as it did pre-pregnancy *in just two weeks*. The message was: Hey, you're supposed to get your old body back immediately.

Why is there so much pressure from society for we women to return to our 'old selves?' Because the truth is that our 'old selves' are nowhere to be found once we become mothers. Everything about our lives shifts—our priorities, our capacity for love, even our shoe sizes. Seriously, no one told me my feet would grow too big for my shoes.

There is no 'old self.' Instead, each of us are faced with a new version of ourselves, a version we must treat with the same love and lack of judgment we have for our children. We need to be celebrating each other for completing that marathon of pregnancy and birth, and to be gentle and allowing of our bodies by acknowledging the enormous physical and emotional changes we have gone through. There is no perfect body, no perfect way to behave or act or be. Motherhood itself is imperfect.

As a millennial mom, I was under the impression—especially via social media—that, in order to be the perfect mother, I should not only take my children to music class and karate lessons and parks and museums and every birthday party they're invited to, I should also play with them all day. We're told to be their moms, their friends, their entertainers, their cooks, and to make sure they're as smart and talented as possible. It's insane. That is not a job for just one person, as social media would have you believe.

Instead, we, as mothers, need to know that it's okay to ask for help. Social media is a great tool, but why don't we use it to reach out to each other and share information, not only about the surprising changes and uncomfortable feelings of pregnancy—which are completely normal—but about how to empower ourselves as mothers, as women? We need to encourage each other to be conscious of our own happiness and well-being, so that we can be the best we can for ourselves, which will ultimately benefit our children more than any perfect uploaded moment. ”

—**Camila Sodi** Singer, Actress, and Model

# Off Tract V

*My patient, Collette, was dating again after the end of her twenty-five-year marriage...and she was thrilled, so thrilled, in fact, that she had stopped by my office the afternoon her divorce was finalized just to show me the papers! With her two sons grown and in college, she was finally free to announce, "The guy was a dick for twenty-four of the twenty-five years we were married, and the only saving grace is my sons!" Collette was on a "Hello Cupid" rampage, making up for lost time, and having sex like crazy (she promised me she was making sure her dates wore condoms). But she was in my office with an embarrassing problem. "Sex is making me pee!" she said. "And I mean during sex! Please tell me there's something I can do about this."*

Ah, yes, just when you think you've finally reached that pot of gold—in Collette's case, it was intimacy and sex after so many years without—there lies the rub. The irony is that women who are sexually active tend to have more urinary tract infections, commonly known as UTIs, than women who aren't. Sorry about that. But (of course) there are certainly means of prevention as well as treatment depending on the *type* of UTI you are diagnosed with. First things first:

## Urinary Tract Infections (UTIs)

Not surprisingly, a UTI refers to an infection of any part of your urinary system—kidney, ureter, bladder, and urethra. The most common UTIs involve the bladder and urethra and occur mainly in women. In fact, 50–60 percent of women will get UTIs in their lifetime! A quarter of those women will have recurrent UTIs—defined by two recurrences within six months or three UTIs in one year.

Why, you may ask, are these types of infections so prevalent in women?

Well, aside from the amazing things that the female anatomy is set up for, it is also a perfect setup for infections of the bladders. In women, the bladder and its very short "tubing"—called the urethra—sit directly along the length of the vagina. It's through the urethra that urine exits the body, the opening of which is the tiny hole right above the entrance into the vagina. Because of the urethra's close proximity to the vagina, during vaginal intercourse, bacteria from the vagina—as well as the rectum—can easily find its way into the urethra and up to the bladder, causing a urinary tract infection.

When bacteria end up where they should not be, symptoms of a UTI can develop within twenty-four hours of having intercourse. Symptoms include:

* Pain or burning with urination
* An urgency to urinate frequently, but only passing a very small amount of urine
* Pain in the lower belly
* Red, pink, or cloudy urine accompanied by a bad odor
* Pain in the lower back
* Fever and chills
* Nausea and vomiting

Those last three groups of symptoms, however—severe back pain, along with fever, chills, nausea, and vomiting—are usually more common symptoms in kidney or upper urinary tract infections.

Aside from the act of sexual intercourse, there are many other causes of UTIs, including spermicides, frequent antibiotic use, anatomical problems, genetic risks, and menopause.

Small consolation, but at least when a UTI rears its head after sexual intercourse, you can pretty much determine the cause. In any event, you'll want to see your health care provider in order to come up with a course of treatment.

For those women with recurrent UTIs, there are certain factors that increase the risk of recurrence. Those include:

* Menopause—the loss of estrogen causes the vaginal tissue to become thin and dry—a condition formerly known as vulvovaginal atrophy—now referred to as Genitourinary Syndrome of Menopause (GSM). GSM can affect the bladder, too, increasing the risk of recurrent UTIs.
* Regular use of spermicides—which negatively affects the normal pH balance of the vagina, a pH balance that helps prevent UTIs
* Frequent antibiotic use for other medical conditions
* Anatomical problems that prevent the bladder from emptying completely
* Genetic risks—here's where you can blame your mother. If she has or had frequent UTIs than you may be more prone to them as well.

For a start, there are many things you can do to try and prevent UTIs before they're an issue.

## Daily UTI Prevention

* First and foremost, good hygiene, which includes the no-brainers: Always remember to wipe "front to back" to avoid bringing unwanted bacteria from the anus to the vaginal area, and wear underwear with a cotton crotch.

* Stay hydrated! Drink lots of water to help keep urine and any unwanted bacteria moving out of your body quickly. (Current rule of thumb is to drink half an ounce for every pound you weigh, every day, spread throughout the day. So, if you're 130 pounds, that means sixty-five ounces daily.)
* Avoid using feminine products that use perfumes and other irritating chemicals that bring disruptive bacteria. And please don't douche!
* Probiotics have gotten mixed reviews as there are no true studies as to their efficacy, but they can't hurt.
* Avoid spermicides.
* Avoid frequent antibiotic use.
* Menopausal women may want to consider vaginal hormonal estrogen therapy.
* D-Mannose—a simple sugar found in many fruits, and which also occurs naturally in some cells in the body—has been shown to prevent or treat UTIs and is available as an oral supplement.
* Uqora—an effective natural drink with Vitamins C, B6, Magnesium, Calcium, Potassium, and D-Mannose—helps flush away from the bladder bacteria that put you at risk for a UTI.
* Include daily doses of Vitamin C—a potent antioxidant that may help to protect against bacteria building up in your bladder, which increases your risk of a UTI. Vitamin C should *not,* however, be used to *treat* a UTI, since it will not be effective at killing the bacteria responsible for the infection.
* Try cranberry juice (hold the Vodka!). Maybe you thought this easy form of prevention was an old wives'

tale, or maybe it was advice your grandmother gave you about when you first started having sex (which means that you have a very hip granny), but there is some truth to the effects of drinking cranberry juice on a regular basis. Some studies report that women who follow such a regimen have fewer visits to their doctors and less incidence of recurrent UTIs. The reason for this may be that cranberry juice (or tablets) makes urine more acidic, which prevents harmful bacterial from building up and sticking to the walls of the bladder. [Of course, there are other medical studies with conflicting evidence regarding the efficacy of cranberries as a reliable source of prevention]. Whether or not you decide to include cranberry juice in your daily diet, remember that it is a means of prevention, not treatment.

### *Urinary Tract Infections After Sex*

There are some methods of preventing UTIs that are specifically geared toward those infections resulting from sexual intercourse. They are:

* Remember to pee *after* sex. That way, you help remove any bacteria that might have made their way into the urethra and bladder. It used to be recommended to women to urinate before having sexual intercourse in order to avoid UTIs, but now we know this is a misconception. Peeing *before* doesn't help *prevent* UTIs; rather, it's after the act when we need unwanted bacteria to leave the body. A general rule of thumb, even when you're not feeling the urge to urinate, is to try

to pee every two to three hours or when you *first* feel the urge. Do not hold in your urine for long periods of time! (Pull into that rest stop on long trips, despite the groans from your passengers—they're not the ones who'll be suffering at the end of your road trip!)

* The cleaner you and your partner's genitals are the better. It should go without saying (but I'll say it anyway) that part of pre-sex cleaning for you and your partner must include washing hands and nails, especially if those hands will be having any contact with the genital area (which I imagine they would be, right?).
* Avoid excessive saliva, spermicides, and lubricants in the genital area.
* Avoid using a diaphragm, vaginal sponge, menstrual cup, and sex toys if you are *prone* to UTIs.
* For women in menopause, vaginal estrogen can help hydrate and moisturize the vagina, making the tissue less prone to infection.

### *Treatment of UTIs*

Sometimes it can be tricky to know if you even have a UTI, since symptoms can be subtle and atypical, but, if you have any inkling that something is up *down there*, see your health care provider to rule out a potentially dangerous UTI.

For uncomplicated UTIs and bladder infections—that is, infections that do not include more advanced symptoms, such as fever and lower back pain—a three-to-seven-day course of antibiotics remains the typical treatment option.

For more severe infections—which may include the aforementioned fever, lower back pain, nausea, or vomiting—intravenous antibiotic treatment along with hospitalization may be necessary.

For women with recurrent infections, daily preventative measures in tandem with preventative medications—including low dose antibiotics—are often prescribed.

*Harriet is a widow whose days are brimming with activity. She spends her mornings either playing doubles on the tennis court with girlfriends or rounds of three-par golf at her local public course. A proud "bubbe" of four grandchildren, she takes care of those children Monday, Wednesday, and Friday afternoons while her daughter works. Tuesdays and Thursdays for the past twenty-five years, she has been a proud volunteer at Providence St. John's Breast Center. Harriet would often call my nurse, Dani, with a complaint of painful urination and pressure sensation in her bladder area, which she assumed was a bladder infection. Since anything that got in the way of Harriet's busy schedule was usually a thing to be ignored, she would also say, "And, Dani, I am way too busy to come in for a urine culture. Would you please just ask Dr. Sherry to call in a prescription?" A prescription would be called in and this same conversation would be repeated every other month. When Harriet finally came in, at my insistence, it turned out that she never had a bladder infection to begin with. What she had had was Interstitial Cystitis—an annoying copycat.*

## Interstitial Cystitis or Bladder Pain Syndrome (IC/BPS)

Interstitial Cystitis (or bladder pain syndrome) looks and acts like a UTI, and certainly feels a helluva lot like one, but it's not.

IC/BPS is a painful, common, and completely under-diagnosed bladder condition affecting up to nearly 7 percent of women. The American Urological Association (AUA) defines IC/BPS as "an unpleasant sensation (pain, pressure, or discomfort) perceived to be related to the urinary bladder, associated with lower urinary tract symptoms of more than six weeks duration, in the absence of infection or other identifiable causes."

Unfortunately, no one knows the exact causes of IC/BPS, but there are a few theories. The one which makes the most sense has to do with the disruption of the protective layer of the bladder, giving certain irritants—which happen to be swimming around in the area—easier access to the nerves and muscles of the bladder, causing discomfort and pain, not unlike that of a UTI.

### *Diagnosis of IC/BPS*

In order for your health care giver to make a proper diagnosis, they will need an accurate history of symptoms. This includes keeping track of the specific location and type of pain you may be experiencing, especially since there is a laundry list of the various possible causes of pelvic pain—which include endometriosis, IBS, fibromyalgia, or recurrent UTIs. Specifics are key in diagnosing IC/BPS, which means being your own best detective in recording the details of your symptoms. Also, urinary tests, which will return positive for UTIs, will prove negative for infection if a woman has IC.

## Off Tract V

### *Treatment of IC/BPS*

No one treatment of IC/BPS works for all sufferers but, since the symptoms are caused by nerve pain, **nerve blocks** with medication may be prescribed as treatment. Physical therapy is another option, as is bladder medication, which is placed directly into the bladder, weekly, for up to eight weeks in order to jump-start treatment.

Most treatments, however, are aimed at simply controlling IC/BPS, the most effective of which includes dietary restrictions. I'm sorry to say that many of our favorite foods (at least mine) are triggers for women with IC. In fact, these food favorites have identified as triggers for up to 90 percent of women diagnosed with IC. So, without further ado, I give you the following culprits to be avoided if you are diagnosed with IC/BPS:

* Coffee
* Tea
* Chocolate
* Alcohol
* Spicy foods
* Citrus
* Tomatoes
* Artificial sweeteners

I know. Why is it always coffee, chocolate, and alcohol? (That's a rhetorical question for the ages.)

In addition to dietary awareness, helpful lifestyle changes include relaxation techniques, efforts to minimize stress, low-impact exercises, warm Sitz baths, loose clothing, bladder training, and monitoring of fluid intake.

In any event, the treatment for IC is ongoing and may last weeks or months (and beyond).

Since symptoms of IC/BPS are wide-ranging and varying in their severity, IC/BPS may be tough to treat. However, the one therapy that most health care givers can agree on is the reduction of stress. In fact, several studies have been done involving a treatment course of mindfulness-based stress reduction.

On that note, mindfulness—the zeitgeist of our millennium—can definitely serve to help conquer, if not ease, whatever ails you. Believe me, it's worth a try. At least after you've made that initial visit to your preferred health care giver. Don't be like Harriet. Make that appointment. And then... Om.

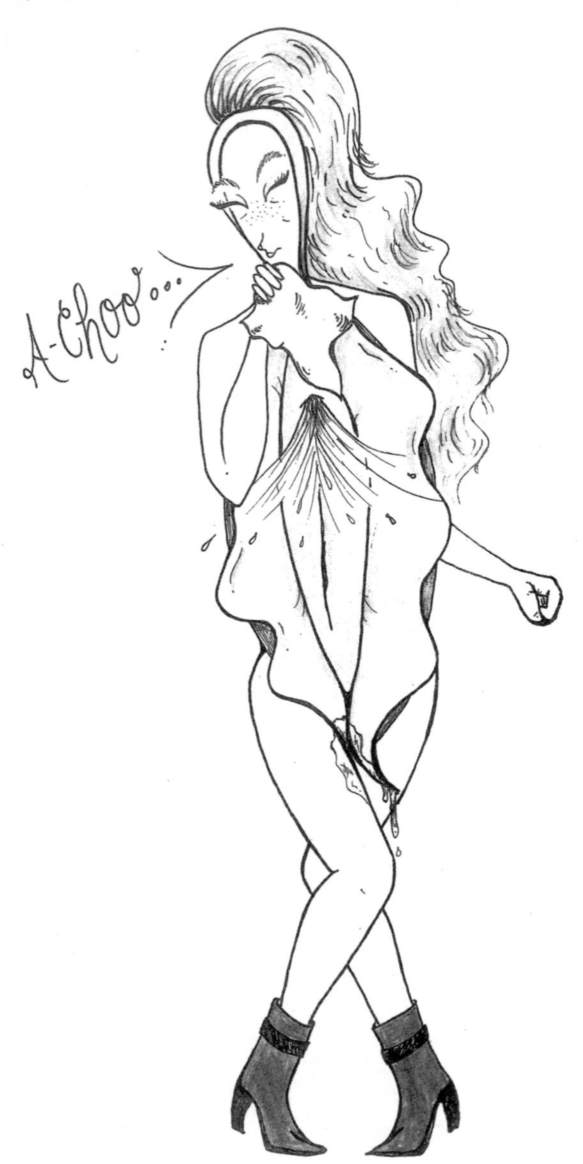
A-Choo...

CHAPTER 5

# V leaky

"When it comes to our health and well-being as women, I've learned that it's important to take the reins ourselves, even though it may seem antithetical to the ways in which we were brought up.

I know this first hand, as I was raised by hippie parents, who, when it came to health decisions, opted more for naturopaths than general practitioners. That is okay for some ailments, but definitely not all.

When I was fourteen, my mother was diagnosed with breast cancer. When it proved inoperable, she chose a path of Eastern medicine for her treatment over a more modern Western one. As hard as she fought, she lost her battle against the disease two years later when she was only forty-two. All the advances in cutting-edge treatments and the new skills of modern kick-ass doctors make me wonder: If she was diagnosed today, would she still be with us?

That was my first introduction to the scary C word. On my mother's side of the family, there has been an aunt diagnosed with breast cancer (who survived) as well as a cousin who died of ovarian cancer at sixteen.

Needless to say, I evolved into somewhat of a hypochondriac. Due to my family history, I scheduled my first mammogram at twenty-three—far younger than the recommended age forty baseline—and have since alternated regular mammograms with breast MRIs.

Fortunately, I also found a gynecologist that didn't make less of my concerns—in fact, one who shared my belief in prevention and testing based on family history, and the pursuit of healthy living as the ultimate best revenge. Not only did that same gynecologist deliver both my babies—after difficult pregnancies and bed rest for months with both—she was a compassionate fount of knowledge every step of the way.

After the birth of my second child, once I'd finished breastfeeding, she supported my choice to do the BART and BRCA tests to find out whether I was positive for the genetic factors most commonly related to female cancers. Truly, I was bracing myself for a double mastectomy, but fortunately my tests proved to be negative.

Not only has that gynecologist, Dr. Sherry Ross, been a true champion for me since we met, she has supplemented my knowledge of women's health issues a thousand-fold.

With all her positivity, instilling in me the idea that testing and self-care are your best weapons in maintaining your health (and happiness), I feel very lucky to have Dr. Sherry in my life. Who knows? One day she may even save it! ”

—**Rachel Roberts** Model and Actress

# Leaky V

*Janice, a lanky forty-seven-year-old supermom of four, comes to see me from her home in Topanga Canyon, always bearing home-grown vegetables from her garden. I'm proud to say that I've delivered all four of her children, but just barely, because she spent most of her labor at home chanting and breathing with her doula—I love that she enlisted the help of a doula, but I also love that she chose to deliver in the safety of a hospital setting. With each child, her labors became progressively faster, so that, by the fourth child, the baby was already crowning when she pulled up to the hospital! Not long after her last child was born, she showed up for a routine exam. Instead of her usual warm smile, she greeted me with tears. Before I could ask what was wrong, she started telling me about how she was peeing in her pants while laughing or running after her kids or having sex with her husband. She said she ignored it at first, but that the "leaking" had gotten progressive worse. Needless to say, she was desperate for answers and solutions.*

Does any of this sound familiar to you (except maybe for the vegetable garden and four kids)? Have you ever been in the midst of jogging, bending, a fit of laughter, or sex and found yourself *leaking*? Have you experienced that horrifying sensation of a warm liquid drip down your thigh and thought: WTF?! Chances are, if it happened at home, you may have simply managed the situation and put it at the back of your mind; but what about the time it happened at that cocktail party, or while grocery shopping or running after your toddler in Target? Worse yet, you remember the time your bladder gave way at the height of a passionate lovemaking session?

Not surprisingly, it seems that problems related to loss of urine remain as taboo as many other vagina-related issues. Sure, losing urine during the most mundane (or extraordinary) activities may be embarrassing or difficult to admit, but, more importantly, it may be the result of an underlying physical condition—one that can be remedied. Certainly, making sanitary pads a part of your daily wardrobe should be a very last resort.

So, if you've said on more than one occasion, "It's so funny I peed my pants!" and have, literally, meant it, you are in good company. The American Academy of Physicians (AAP) found that 50 percent of women between the ages of forty and sixty, and almost 75 percent of women over the age of seventy-five suffer from loss of urine, medically known as Genuine Stress Urinary Incontinence, or GSUI. To no one's surprise, stress incontinence affects twice as many women as it does men—which may be why drug manufacturers aren't scrambling to make a little blue pill to address *that* particular issue.

## GSUI (Genuine Stress Urinary Incontinence)

Urinary incontinence, which is classified as either stress or urge incontinence—occurs when (surprise, surprise) one loses urine. With GSUI, over time, the urethra—the tube through which urine leaves the bladder and is conveyed out of the body—weakens with physical distress or trauma, or simple wear and tear.

Stress incontinence is basically the result of weakened pelvic floor muscles, those muscles that support the bladder and the urethra and are thereby most susceptible to the wear and tear of childbirth, obesity, chronic coughing, sneezing, and constipation, or regular high-impact exercises. Older women,

women who have had vaginal deliveries, obese women, and women who have undergone hysterectomies are typically the most prone to stress incontinence. One may even inherit GSUI—which means that you may be predisposed to urinary incontinence because Aunt Selma had it first! Any activity that increases abdominal pressure can bring on stress incontinence, especially if your bladder is full—coughing, sneezing, laughing, exercising, heavy lifting, walking, standing up, getting out of the car, or having sex.

Aside from being embarrassing and isolating, stress incontinence may limit one's ability to perform typical daily activities and exercise. Often, women suffering from GSUI must wear pads or diapers to get through the day—humiliating, for sure, but also a cause for perpetual "diaper rash" of the vulva. The emotional distress alone may be enough to keep a woman from social interactions, sexual intimacy, and normal daily routines.

Although GSUI can happen to any woman at any time in her life, there are certain factors that may exacerbate its onset, such as (not surprisingly):

* Alcohol
* Caffeine
* Soda
* Chocolate
* Artificial Sweeteners
* Cigarette smoking
* Obesity
* Urinary Tract Infections
* Complications of Diabetes
* Medications causing frequent or excessive urine production

Urge incontinence is different (and less common) than stress incontinence in that the cause of urine loss is unrelated to any specific activity. Urge incontinence often occurs as a result of an overactive bladder muscle. However, for some unlucky women, stress and urge incontinence can occur together.

## Diagnosis of GSUI

In the case of regular loss of urine or incontinence, you're going to need to keep a diary of your urination habits, including how often you urinate and how much fluid you drink, in order to start to identify the problem.

Your health care provider may start with a pelvic exam, urine analysis, and culture. They may then proceed with a post-void residual—which is a test that determines whether there is residual urine in your bladder after peeing—or they may refer you to a urologist for further testing and accurate diagnosis, after which they can select a treatment plan.

In extreme causes, urodynamic testing, typically performed by a urologist, may be necessary. This type of testing may involve a series of procedures measuring the strength of your bladder and the rate of voiding under bladder and rectal pressures. Your urologist may suggest a cystoscopy, a procedure involving the insertion of a hollow tube, equipped with a lens, through your urethra and into your bladder.

## Treatment of GSUI

### *Lifestyle*

Treatment options for women who suffer from loss of urine may vary, depending on how disruptive your loss of urine is in your everyday life, but basic lifestyle changes may make all the difference in the world. Those changes include:

* Limiting fluid intake, especially after dinner!
* Trying biofeedback to help identify your pelvic floor muscles in order to make sure that you are contracting them correctly.
* Emptying your bladder regularly and avoid "holding it in" too long!
* Controlling asthma and other lung problems with the right medications.
* Figuring out what your food triggers may be and avoiding them.
* Stop smoking!
* Keeping your BMI under 30
* Don't strain with bowel movements, and, to that end, avoid constipation
* And [drum roll, please] practicing the almighty Pelvic Floor Muscle Training, better known as Kegels, which I'll get to a bit later.
* As a last resort (temporary or not), don't hesitate to use incontinence products such as absorbent pads, adult diapers, and hand-help urinals to prevent embarrassing accidents.

### *Medications and Devices*

Sadly, there aren't many dependable remedies without annoying side effects you can store in your medicine cabinet to treat stress incontinence.

Duloxetine (brand name, Cymbalta) a drug used to treat depression, is believed to also aid in treatment of stress incontinence, but it hasn't yet been approved for that purpose in the United States.

A vaginal pessary, which is a soft, removable device in the shape of a ring, is sometimes used to lessen the symptoms of urine loss by keeping the bladder in its normal anatomical position. Pessaries are often used as an alternative to surgical procedures. However, not all women are good candidates for a vaginal pessary, due to age or other medical problems. Much like that good old-fashioned diaphragm, pessaries need to be removed and cleaned regularly to avoid vaginal infections.

Surprisingly enough, incontinence has been known to be treated with Botox injections—go ahead, try to imagine Botox for the bladder—even though the FDA has not officially approved this type of treatment. In this process Botox is injected on both sides of the bladder to keep the detrusor muscles from suddenly contracting and leading to urination. Medical studies show that Botox can improve symptoms by 90 percent over a one-year period. Just be sure you get that Botox injection from a trained urologist and not your favorite cosmetician!

Urethral bulking, another minimally invasive procedure used to treat incontinence, is useful when the cause is due to intrinsic sphincter deficiency—a fancy blanket term referring to some type of urethral weakness. It involves injections of "bulking agents," which may include collagen and water-based gels into the wall of the urethra in order to ensure a watertight seal—think: caulking for the urethra. This is usually an option for women who aren't fit enough for surgery and anesthesia, or for those who aren't done with childbearing.

### *Surgery*

As a last resort, surgery is often the answer. Sling surgery, the most common procedure to treat urinary stress incontinence, involves creating a "sling" out of mesh or human tissue, which then acts to support the urethra and help keep it closed when laughing, sneezing, coughing—you name it—when you do anything that shouldn't require simultaneous peeing!

Along that vein, Colposuspension is another surgical treatment option used to ensure long-term treatment of stress incontinence. The procedure, which is performed under general anesthetic, involves making an incision in the abdomen in order to lift the bladder neck upward and stitch it into this lifted position.

Urge incontinence can also be treated through electrical stimulation of some of the key nerves that control bladder functioning. This procedure, which is usually done for severe cases, involves surgically implanting a device to stimulate the nerves involved in urination in order to make the bladder behave properly.

For more complicated types of urinary incontinence, there are other more advanced surgical treatment options that may be discussed with a urologist.

Last, and certainly not least, what I consider to be the Holy Grail for strong pelvic and vaginal muscles [drum roll, please]...

### *Kegels*

Kegel exercises are the most simple and effective way to strengthen those pelvic floor muscles—muscles that support the uterus, bladder, and bowels, which, in turn, control bladder and bowel function. I tell even my youngest patients: You are never too young to start those Kegels!

There are many reasons for weakened pelvic floor muscles—pregnancy, childbirth, aging, weight gain—but the results of those weakened muscles are not discriminating. When your pelvic floor muscles are weak, pelvic organs can begin to drop, creating a bulge into your vagina. When this occurs, it is called pelvic organ prolapse. Symptoms from a prolapse may range from uncomfortable pelvic pressure to urine leakage, which is where those Kegel exercises come into play. Kegels can actually help delay and even prevent pelvic organ prolapse and its related symptoms.

So how does one "do" a Kegel exercise?

First, you must identify your pelvic floor muscles. The easiest way to do this is to try and stop your flow of urine mid-pee, so to speak, and hold it for a few seconds, then relax. Repeat; pee and hold. Those muscles contracting? Those are your Kegel muscles.

Another way to identify your Kegel muscles is to insert your first two fingers into your vagina and squeeze your pelvic muscles as if you are holding urine. You should feel your vagina tighten and your pelvic floor move upward. Relax your muscles and feel your pelvic floor return to the starting position.

Once you've identified your Kegel muscles, you can begin your exercises. First, empty your bladder, and then sit or lie down. Contract your pelvic floor muscles—as you did when you peed—hold the contraction for five seconds, and then relax for five seconds. Try it four or five times in a row. Work your way up to keeping the muscles contracted for ten seconds at a time, relaxing for fifteen seconds between contractions.

Start with fifteen contractions daily, gradually increasing to fifty (yes, fifty, we're talking about keeping your pelvic organs where they were intended to be!). I promise, if you do your Kegels faithfully, you'll notice a benefit to your pelvic floor strength in just eight to twelve weeks. With diligence (and patience) 40 to 60 percent of women see an improvement in their symptoms of loss of urine after three months. Talk about zero cost and priceless results!

If you are looking for an easy, painless, and silent partner in doing your Kegel exercises, you can slip on a pair of INNOVO® shorts. This innovative FDA-cleared solution delivers perfect, pain-free muscle stimulations to strengthen the muscles in the pelvic floor and treat the root cause of Leaky V, not just the symptoms. Think TENS unit for the pelvic floor!

I can't say enough about the practice of doing Kegels, and the very cool and convenient thing about them is that you can perform them almost anywhere, anytime, without anyone being the wiser. Please make this Holy Grail of vagina care a permanent part of your daily routine.

For those of you who need more convincing, I give you the argument of....

### *Kegels and Sex*

Exactly. Kegel exercises can also make sexual intercourse more enjoyable for you *and* your partner. If you do your Kegels during vaginal intercourse, the muscles contract on the penis, enhancing *his* sexual experience, just as a Kegel performed while trying to orgasm yourself will only enhance *your* orgasm—and who doesn't love that?

What I want to stress is that no woman should ever be embarrassed to talk about a leaky V. The time to talk about it is now, before, during, and after its occurrence.

In fact, new guidelines in the screening of urinary incontinence have recently been announced. According to the Women's Preventative Service Initiative, these guidelines recommend that all women should undergo annual screening for urinary incontinence beginning in adolescence, and that clinicians should refer their patients for further evaluation and treatment when appropriate. This recommendation will help identify women at risk or those already suffering from urinary incontinence in order to begin early treatment strategies.

Kegel exercises, along with the maintenance of a healthy body weight early in life are two of the easiest, no-brainer precautions to help avoid challenging medications, surgical procedures, and shocking medical bills down the road due to urinary incontinence.

If you're already suffering from some kind of urinary incontinence, whether it seems manageable or extreme, keep a diary of how often you are peeing, how much liquid you are consuming, and when. This will be helpful in identifying if you are just drinking a ton of water or you have problem with a weak bladder.

Keep track of the circumstances and well as your emotional state. Are you losing urine with exercise? Laughter? Sex? How often are you getting up in the middle of the night to pee? Do you feel like your insides are coming out of your vagina? Are you avoiding social interactions as result of loss of urine? Is it resulting in depression or anxiety?

## Leaky V

This may not be your ideal journal, but it can certainly help in determining a strategy for your leaky V. Trust me, you are in good company!

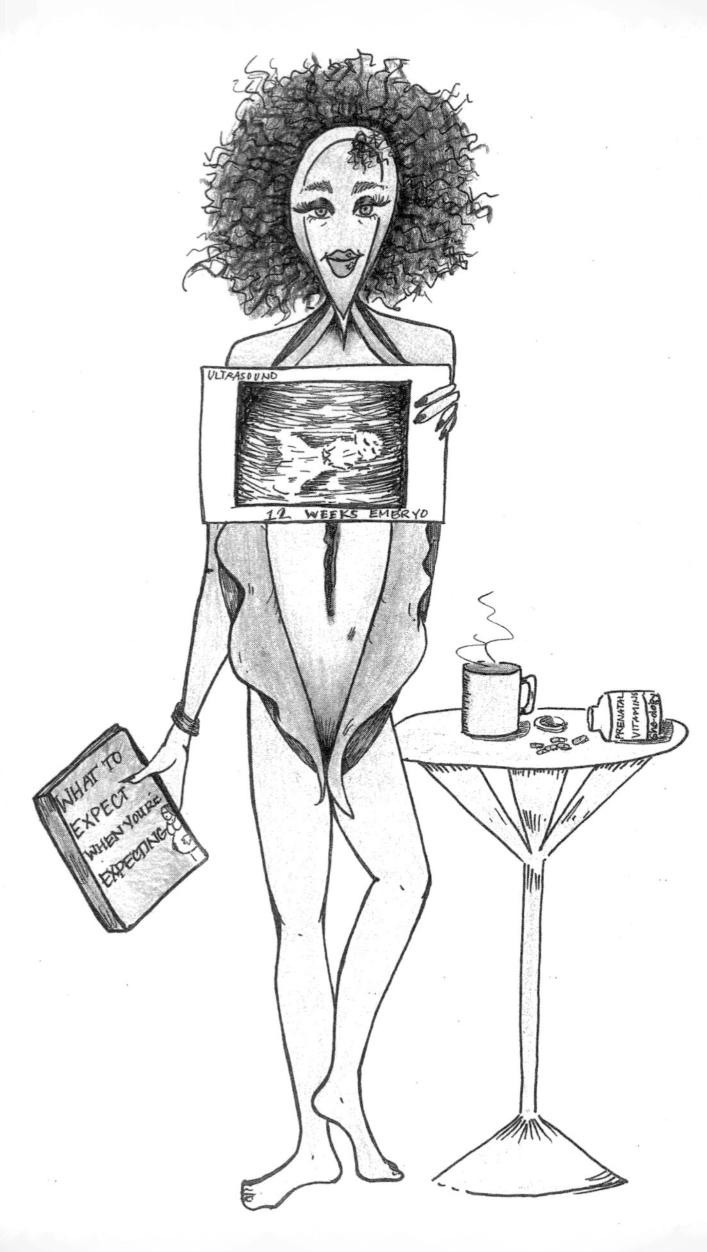
ULTRASOUND
12 WEEKS EMBRYO
WHAT TO EXPECT WHEN YOU'RE EXPECTING
PRENATAL VITAMINS

CHAPTER 6

# pregnant

"I always knew I wanted to be a mother, but I also knew it wasn't something I could force. Fortunately, I found myself with the person I wanted to spend my life with, and I became pregnant *while* we were planning our wedding. I was loved and supported and ready, so the timing was right.

I was born code blue—which is the term used when a baby isn't breathing—so the idea of not having my baby delivered by an experienced doctor, in a hospital, seemed crazy to me. It was important then to find a doctor whose confidence and knowledge was undeniable. No surprise, the doctor I chose turned out to be Dr. Sherry.

Having total confidence in my doctor definitely helped me relax about my pregnancy. Avoiding most of the books people sent me about being pregnant helped as well, by keeping me from getting in my head about all the 'shoulds' and worries and things that could go wrong. Trusting my intuition was also key—I'm pretty intuitive to begin with, since it's the 'muscle' I work out the most as an actor—so, during my pregnancy, I continued to trust that intuition and did what felt right *for me.*

The one book I did read was by an economist who talked about how to be a chill pregnant person in every sense of the way, and to not get trapped by following blanket rules. That especially gave me the freedom to relax and trust my intuition. Of course, like everyone else, I'd worry a little before each checkup, but I didn't dwell on the worry.

I also enjoyed being pregnant (I may be one of the few). I'm fine being in bed and resting, getting into that cozy zone. In the first trimester, when I felt chronically jet-lagged, I just slept whenever I could. And I lived in my bathtub the last trimester—kind of a human prune.

The difficult part of my pregnancy came when I found out that my baby was breach, which meant my plans for a vaginal birth were done. I was so disappointed because I'd been looking forward to that experience, but my kid just did not want to move into the right position. That scared me in a way I hadn't been until then.

I'd never had major surgery, so I was far less afraid of giving birth than I was of the surgery itself. But everyone involved in the delivery was so calm. They'd done it a million times. They were like, *Here we go, we're gonna wheel you in and get your baby out!* After it was over, and my baby was safely delivered, all I could think was 'Thank God for modern medicine, or we both probably would've died.'

Later, I asked Dr. Sherry about the trend of saving one's placenta to eat. She was her usual straightforward self in giving me all the latest info, but added, 'The science isn't there to back it all up, so it's questionable, especially if it's not boiled right.'

I thought, 'Thank God I have a doctor I trust.' ”

—**Kirsten Dunst** Actress

## Pregnant V

"Going through my wife's pregnancy was an extraordinary experience, not to mention an *education*. I wanted to be in the room during conception. I mean, sure, I was a little light-headed, but I got through it. To be in the room during the delivery, though, was another story. I was not good with blood, but I decided to be there because I was a team player and, more importantly, I didn't want to be discovered as the coward I was. I agreed to provide music for the event, so I downloaded a bunch of songs on my iPod and figured I could avoid any unpleasant occurrences by focusing on my playlist.

I arrived home late one night to find my wife in labor. Since her contractions weren't close enough together, it wasn't time to go to the hospital, but, by four a.m., I suggested we make our move. I didn't want to run the risk of getting stuck in traffic and having our baby on the freeway.

We headed off to St. John's Hospital in Santa Monica. There was no one on the road. I was actually able to see pavement in front of my car for the first time ever driving in Los Angeles. We cruised along the coast as the majestic waves of the Pacific Ocean crashed onto the shore and the sun peered over the Santa Monica Mountains. I looked down at my wife's belly and thought: This is such a miracle—NO TRAFFIC!

When we arrived, I hooked my iPod up to my speakers and Dr. Ross hooked my wife up to her monitors. We both had our jobs. It's what we trained for. Before long, a very calm Dr. Ross asked me if I would like to help. 'Absolutely,' I said. 'I'm working the iPod.'

'No, I mean, would you like to help with the delivery?'

*No! Absolutely not!* That's what I should've said, but, because I'm a people-pleaser and dislike confrontation I said, 'Sure. That would be a great experience.' She then handed me latex gloves, which meant something was going to get wet and it better not be the iPod. She instructed me to hold my wife's left leg up in the air—which is how

I got into this position in the first place! I was frustrated because I couldn't hold her leg and work the iPod at the same time. In hindsight, I should've hired a D.J. I would have had him hold my wife's leg and I could have done my job properly.

Then everything happened so quickly. After the baby's head came out, Dr. Ross asked if I wanted to pull out the rest of it.

No! Not a chance! But, again, because I wanted to be liked, I said, 'Sure, what an opportunity.'

I pulled on the head but nothing else came out. It seemed like its neck was just extending longer and longer. I told Dr. Ross I was afraid I was going to pull the baby's head off. She said that wouldn't happen. I said, 'Okay, but, if it does, I'm going to be very angry with you!'

Up until then, we didn't know what the sex of the baby was. We wanted it to be a surprise. But you know how it is; you don't care if it's a boy or a girl, just as long as it…*has a penis.* I finally gave a good tug and it slipped right out and I saw that it did have a penis! It was really the only time in my life I was excited to see one—other than my own. Dr. Ross then asked me if I wanted to cut the umbilical cord. At this point, I was thinking, 'Sheez! Doesn't anyone wanna work around here? Why do I have to do everything? Do you wanna come to our house and cut the grass and wash the dishes? You can tell everyone you helped.' But I took the scissors and 'snip-snip.' No big deal. In hindsight, it was a great experience, for all of us. In fact, a couple hours later, I went across the hall and delivered two more babies. ”

—**Kevin Nealon** Comedian and Actor

## Meet the Pregnant V: A Personality Unto Itself!

Let's just say that my working title for this particular chapter was Super V [think: big, red V on a yellow and blue background, cape, Anthropomorphic Superhero Vagina...okay, stop me here]. You get the picture. The point being that a pregnant vagina truly exemplifies the seemingly superhuman capabilities of women. A whole host of changes are in store for your pregnant V, some of which may make your vagina wholly unrecognizable in color, size, feeling, and smell. If you ever thought your vagina had its own personality *pre-pregnancy,* get ready for your fabulous V as it accommodates a growing human, twenty-four/seven, without a break.

To begin with—for the record—I've compiled a list of the most common questions I hear from pregnant women. Not surprisingly, in the number one spot:

### *1. How Much Weight Do I Really Have to Gain During Pregnancy?*

Many women dread the answer to this question, but the amount of weight you should gain in pregnancy can depend on a number of important factors:

* Are you pregnant with one (singleton) or two (twins) or three (triplets) babies?
* What is your age and what is your pre-pregnancy weight?
* Do you have any additional medical conditions, such as gestational diabetes or hypertension, that will affect the overall recommended weight gain?

Pregnancy is not a situation whereby the more weight you gain, the healthier your baby. On the contrary, excessive weight gain sets the baby up for future health problems. The days of "eating for two" are long gone. The more you eat and the more weight you gain during pregnancy won't make the baby sleep better at night, breastfeed easier, crawl sooner, or, for that matter, get into your local private school more easily. In fact, a woman of average weight before pregnancy should gain twenty-five to thirty-five pounds during pregnancy.

In order to gain the "right" amount of weight gain during pregnancy, you must incorporate a healthy and balanced diet so that your baby receives all the nutrients he or she needs to grow at a healthy rate. A recent study showed 48 percent of women gain more weight, 21 percent gain below, and 32 percent gain within the recommended recommendation. In general, you will need to consume up to 100 to 400 more calories a day, depending on what trimester you are in, in order to meet the needs of your growing baby. Basically, you should gain about two to four pounds during your first three months of pregnancy, and one pound a week thereafter.

Guidelines for weight gain during a singleton pregnancy are as follows:

* Underweight women (BMI < 18.5), 28–40 pounds.
* Normal weight women (BMI 18.5–24.9), 25–35 pounds.
* Overweight women (BMI 25–29.9), 15–25 pounds.
* Obese women (BMI 30 or higher), 11–20 pounds.

The good news is that the majority of women will return to their normal body weight within nine months of having their baby.

## 2. *When Should I Feel Fetal Movement?*

Most women feel the beginnings of fetal movement before twenty-one weeks of gestation. In a first pregnancy, this can occur at around eighteen to twenty-one weeks, and, in subsequent pregnancies, it can occur as early as fifteen to sixteen weeks into pregnancy. Early fetal movement is felt most commonly when a woman is sitting or lying quietly and concentrating on her body. A woman may also feel fetal movement after eating or after *drinking a sugary beverage*—which ought to give anyone pause about sugary foods and beverages.

## 3. *How Can I Prevent Stretch Marks?*

*I like stretch marks*—said no women ever on any planet. Those pink, reddish, or purplish indented streaks that often appear on the belly, breasts, upper arms, buttocks, and thighs are a bane of any pregnant woman. Unfortunately, stretch marks cannot be prevented, since they are genetically determined, which means that, if your mom got them, especially during pregnancy, you probably will too.

Stretch marks usually occur when you gain or lose weight quickly. Despite their marketing, *special creams and gels* rarely make much of a difference in the appearance of such marks. Although stretch marks will fade with time—becoming silvery white or red—they rarely disappear completely. The good news is that, once pregnancy is over, you can manage your stretch marks using the newest laser treatments.

## 4. *What Foods Should I Avoid During Pregnancy?*

Raw fish, such as sushi, is not recommended in pregnancy, since it can carry certain bacteria and parasites. Mercury, unfortunately found in a lot of fish around the world, is very toxic and can cause problems to the fetus and to the newborn nursing infant. Shark, grouper, Chilean sea bass, halibut, swordfish, king mackerel, tuna, and tilefish have been found to contain some of the highest mercury levels in seafood, and therefore pose the greatest risk in pregnant women.

However, a pregnant woman can safely eat twelve ounces per week of a variety of fish found to be low in mercury. Those fish usually include shrimp, canned light tuna, scallops, oysters, squid, and salmon.

The foods listed below should be avoided in order to decrease the risk of food-borne illness caused by the bacteria Listeriosis. Listeriosis is thirteen times more common to occur in pregnant women and causes serious complications to both woman and baby.

* Unpasteurized milk and foods made with unpasteurized milk, including soft cheeses such as feta, queso blanco, queso fresco, Camembert, Brie, or blue-veined cheeses, unless the label says: "made with pasteurized milk"
* Hot dogs, luncheon meats, and cold cuts, unless they are heated
* Refrigerated pate and meats spreads
* Refrigerated smoked seafood
* Raw and undercooked beef, pork, poultry, and eggs

Also, be aware that Salmonella and E. coli can be passed through undercooked meat, poultry, and eggs.

* **Drinking coffee while pregnant.** Sadly, for many coffee lovers, caffeine in large quantities has been shown to

cause miscarriages during the first trimester and may, with excessive consumption, decrease the baby's birth weight. That said, consuming less than 200mg of caffeine a day—a twelve-ounce cup of coffee—is considered safe for mother and baby.

* **Drinking herbal teas while pregnant.** Drinking two cups of caffeinated tea a day is safe for your growing baby. And the good news is that you can drink as much decaffeinated herbal tea as you want.

### *5. What Is the Best Sleep Position for Me During Pregnancy?*

During pregnancy, normal sleep patterns are completely disrupted. And, while a pregnancy-related sleep disorder is not a specific diagnosis, it has been proposed as a new categorization by the American Sleep Disorder Association. Disruptions such as positional discomfort, contractions, leg cramps, gastric reflux, and frequent urination may be factors leading to disordered sleep patterns.

It is also not uncommon for women to need more (or less) sleep in pregnancy. Typically, the amount of sleep needed is *increased* in the first and second trimester and actually *decreases* in the third trimester. The amount of REM and deeper stage sleep also changes in pregnancy.

Whether you've slept on your back, stomach, or side *before* pregnancy, you may have to find a new sleeping position for optimal health *during* your pregnancy.

In fact, after twenty weeks, because of the *weight* of your growing uterus, it's best to sleep on your right or left side (even better). Sleeping on your back puts additional pressure from the uterus on the vessels supplying blood to the heart, which can cause your blood pressure to drop and make you feel dizzy or lightheaded. Less blood flow *to* the heart means less blood flow *out* of the heart, and less blood flow to the baby, which could ultimately affect its growth. Lying on your back can also cause breathing problems and/or worsening heartburn. I suggest using the three-pillow strategy—one pillow under your head, one between your arms and one placed between your knees—or a full-body pillow for complete body, belly, and limb support.

## *6. What are the Best Forms of Pain Management During a Vaginal Delivery?*

Epidurals have gotten a bad rap—whether via old wives' tales or urban legend. *News flash:* An epidural will *not* cause you to be paralyzed following delivery or experience any permanent nerve damage.

In fact, an epidural is an effective means of blocking pain in the lower part of the body and is safe for you and your baby. An anesthesiologist numbs a pea-sized area of your lower back, and then places a very thin needle into your spinal cord and threads a catheter through it, which will be used to deliver the numbing medication. The needle is then carefully removed, allowing the catheter to stay in place during labor.

Epidurals do a perfect job of relaxing a woman in labor. With an epidural, you do not have the problem of feeling drugged or foggy, as you would have with intravenous sedation. When you are feeling the relentless pain of labor, every muscle in your body tenses up, including your uterus, but, once you are comfortable and pain-free from an epidural, your body becomes relaxed enough to allow the natural process of labor to happen more easily.

If the relaxation effect provided by an epidural relaxes the uterus to the point that it slows down uterine contractions, labor may be slowed down as well. In this case, the medication Pitocin can safely increase the frequency and intensity of uterine contractions. When it's time to start pushing out the baby, an epidural is turned off to allow you to feel the rectal sensation in order to push most effectively.

Lighter-dosed epidurals, called "walking epidurals," are used for those women who prefer less sedation and more mobility during labor.

Complications of an epidural occur only in about 1 percent of women and may include postpartum headaches.

For those women that elect a C-Section, a onetime dose of a shorter-acting spinal anesthesia is typically given. If you are in labor with an epidural and need a C-Section, the medication used to numb you during this surgical procedure is given through the catheter already in place.

As for laughing your way through pregnancy: Laughing gas, also known as happy gas, is not a new fad in helping to take the edge off the agony of painful contractions—in fact, laughing gas has been used for pain relief since the 1800s, especially by dentists. In the 1950s, nitrous oxide, which is the active ingredient in laughing gas, was routinely used for women during labor. When epidural anesthesia was introduced in the 1970s, it was found to be a more reliable and effective pain option, although, in Europe, nitrous oxide is regularly used for women in labor.

Usually, a laughing gas "cocktail" of 50 percent nitrous oxide and 50 percent oxygen, laughing gas is delivered through a breathing mask, thereby eliciting a feeling of euphoria and relaxation. Basically, with the cocktail, one becomes less aware of the intensity of the pain experienced during labor. Midwives, in particular, prefer nitrous oxide for a number of reasons:

* Allows patient to move around in labor
* Short acting
* Self-administrated by inhalation
* Effective for mild pain of labor
* Safe alternative option of pain relief for mom and baby
* Easy to use
* Has a euphoric, anti-anxiety, and relaxing effect
* Leaves the body in minutes
* Less expensive than current pain-relief options
* Midwives and other trained medical staff can administer nitrous oxide
* Colorless and nonflammable gas with a slightly sweet odor

Complications of using nitrous oxide during labor may include nausea, vomiting, dizziness, and feelings of lethargy.

Although the benefits seem to far outweigh the few rare complications, a recent study in Anesthesiology 2016 showed that nitrous oxide isn't effective for *extreme* pain, and those women suffering from such pain will ultimately need an epidural for true relief. In other words, nitrous oxide will never replace an epidural as the ideal way to manage labor pain. Truly, the pain of labor is no laughing matter.

### *7. Episiotomies: To Cut or Not to Cut—That Is the Question*

Most women have heard one horror story or another from friends (or friends of friends) or in chat rooms about long painful recoveries from episiotomies, so the first question I hear about that particular procedure is: "Do you automatically cut an episiotomy?" I reassure my patients that an episiotomy is no longer the *standard* of practice—it is no longer *routine*.

It used to be this procedure was done automatically with the intent to make enough room for the baby's head to be delivered with the least amount of damage to the vagina, but now obstetricians find it's no longer *necessary* during a vaginal delivery. In fact, an episiotomy tends to make damage to the vagina worse than a tear. Vaginal tearing is now the more common option and is usually recommended by obstetricians over an episiotomy.

Tearing is not necessarily a given, but there are factors that increase a woman's chance of tearing during childbirth. Those factors include:

* If it's your first baby
* Having a larger-than-normal-size baby
* Vacuum or forceps assisted delivery
* If the baby is being born face-up (occiput posterior)
* Uncontrollable pushing
* Needing to expedite delivery due to fetal distress
* Severe vaginal swelling due to prolonged pushing

Severe tears or extensive episiotomies into the vagina or rectum can cause pelvic floor dysfunction and prolapse, urinary incontinence, fecal incontinence, and sexual dysfunction, including pain with intercourse. However, it's been my experience to allow the vagina to tear naturally during the delivery. The extent of the damage to the vagina seems to be less and the recovery is easier if tearing is allowed to occur. The Mama V—as detailed in my first book *She-ology: The Definitive Guide to Women's Intimate Health. Period.*—has enough to worry about during the first couple weeks without having to deal with the pain and sorrow of an episiotomy repair.

I always reassure my patients that the decision of cutting the vagina or letting the tissue tear naturally is determined at the time of the delivery. The factors determining an episiotomy include how long the woman has been pushing, how large the baby's head is, how swollen the vagina is, and whether there is reason to deliver the baby quickly due to fetal distress. The best interest of mom and baby is first and foremost.

If, indeed, an episiotomy is necessary (for any of the aforementioned reasons) complications may include infection, longer healing time, bleeding, pain at the site of the episiotomy, and future pain with intercourse.

Do yourself and your V a favor and have this "episiotomy or not" conversation with your obstetrician during the third trimester of pregnancy so that you are comfortably aware of what to expect during the vaginal birth of your baby.

You will have more questions and want more answers, believe me, because every woman is different, as is every situation. The changes that happen to your body are real and potentially distressing, but, before you rush into anxiety mode, it's good to be aware of why and how those changes occur, what you might do to ease any discomfort, and when you might want to check in with your health provider.

> *Hanna was in her usual uniform of Gap sweat suit, wild brown hair secured in a ponytail, and a cellphone practically glued to one ear. She was continuously interrupted by her housekeeper, who'd call to say that Hanna's five-year old daughter was not listening...again. Pregnant with her third girl at the ripe old birthing age of forty, Hanna was, by week thirty, clearly done being pregnant.*

*She'd been plagued with varicose veins so severe that it was intensely painful to stand for more than a couple hours. In addition, during this particular visit she complained of vaginal pain and pressure that had her convinced #3 was on her way. "Can't we just deliver this baby?" She said, only half-jokingly. "I am so over it! Just check me into the hospital, hook up an epidural and start the Pitocin. I don't give a shit anymore!" I did a pelvic exam and saw that large, plump veins had taken over the normal structure of her vagina. I explained that her varicose veins were extended all across her vagina, which was the reason for the pain and pressure. I broke out the mirror I use for the purpose of giving my patients a chance to look "down south," and I gave Hanna a glimpse. She was mortified at what she saw, but I assured her that it wasn't uncommon.*

## Vulvar Varicose Veins

We hope and pray we can avoid varicose veins, pregnant or not. When we think of them, they are often the raised roadmaps on our mothers' or grandmothers' *legs*, which is where they are typically found, but varicose veins can also be found in the vulvar area. We refer to them as vulvar varicose veins. Symptoms, such as the ones described by Hanna, include pain and pressure—aside from inducing a great deal of frustration! Go ahead and blame your family for this one because, if you have a family history of varicose veins, you'll be prone to them as well.

Weak veins in the vulvar area become enlarged and swollen as the weight of the growing uterus puts extra pressure on them. These varicose veins are very common in pregnancy, even if they can be difficult to see. At their most severe, vulvar varicose veins can cause pain and bleeding.

In order to prevent varicose veins, or at least help reduce their symptoms, best to:

* Avoid prolonged standing or sitting.
* Wear compression stockings such as a Ted Hose, which reaches to your knee or thigh.
* Elevate your legs one hour, two to three times a day if you must be on your feet a lot during the day.
* Exercise! Not surprisingly, it helps. Aim for three to five times a week for a minimum of thirty minutes.

The good news? Once you have delivered your baby, those vulvar varicose veins will disappear completely or become unnoticeable.

## Yeast and Bacterial Infections

The earliest change you may notice regarding your vagina is an increase in vaginal secretions that appear milky white. You may notice a heavy white discharge, unaccompanied by itching, and wonder if you have a yeast infection. With all the hormonal changes during pregnancy, it is completely normal to experience this kind of discharge. Unless there are other symptoms, such as itching and yellow, green, or red discharge, it is probably normal.

Unfortunately, yeast and bacterial infections are much more common in pregnancy. Since there's more blood flow to the vagina during pregnancy, the normal bacteria that live inside the vagina can be disrupted. This may allow yeast to grow or promote an overgrowth of bacteria, followed by an infection, which can be easily diagnosed with a vaginal culture. If at all in doubt, your obstetrician can do a vaginal culture to be on the safe side.

## Vaginal Bleeding

During pregnancy, vaginal bleeding can be a very concerning symptom, especially depending on the severity. *Spotting/minimal bleeding*—meaning a few drops—is probably nothing to worry about.

*Implantation bleeding* is fairly common occurring in 30 percent of pregnant women and happens around the time you would expect your next period—day twenty-four to twenty-six of your first trimester. The bleeding appears minimal or light, with mild uterine cramping. The main difference between normal implantation bleeding and an abnormal pregnancy is the amount of bleeding you experience and the severity of uterine cramping.

*Mild bleeding* is the light soaking of less than one pad or tampon in three hours, and *moderate bleeding* is characterized by the soaking of more than one pad or tampon in three hours. *Severe bleeding* suggests passing blood clots and soaking through pads or tampons each hour for two or more hours and may be the result of an abnormal pregnancy. If you do have more than spotting, best to contact your physician and describe the degree of bleeding.

Statistics show that, in the first trimester, vaginal bleeding can suggest a miscarriage, although 25 percent of women will normally have spotting or mild bleeding. Of this group, 50 percent will have a normal pregnancy, while the other 50 percent will go on to have a miscarriage. If there is cramping with moderate to severe bleeding, it is more likely than not to be an abnormal pregnancy.

Vaginal bleeding in the third trimester can suggest a problem with the placenta. If the placenta partially or completely covers the cervical outlet, the condition is called a placenta previa. The case of the placenta separating from the uterus is considered an obstetrical emergency, since such a case could be catastrophic to the growing baby.

Whether you're a first-timer or a pregnancy pro, bleeding anytime during pregnancy can be frightening. In my own practice, I want to know if any of my pregnant patients have spotting or bleeding, regardless of the trimester. However, the most likely time to be concerned is if the bleeding is like a heavy period and is accompanied by moderate to severe cramping. Don't hesitate to contact your obstetrician/health care provider immediately if either of those two symptoms occur, separately or together.

## Sex and the Pregnant V

*Linda and her husband, Thomas, were newly married when Linda found herself pregnant. Was it planned? No, but they were truly excited about starting a family. At thirty-three, Linda was that gal at the gym—you'd see her and think: Does she ever take a day off? She was there seven days a week, with her thirty-two-ounce water bottle and high-protein/"good carbs" bar and perfect mane of Dry Bar styled hair. She was fit, attractive, and—one might think—still in the throes of that newlywed stage of sexual desire, but, at her twenty-six-week visit, after eagerly listening to the heartbeat of her son in the ultrasound, she said to me a bit incredulously, "Do women really like to have sex during pregnancy?" That one made me smile. She went on, "I mean, aside from the fact that Thomas is afraid to come near me because he's worried his penis will hurt the baby, I am so not feeling sexy. Truth is that I'd rather order in dinner, stream a movie, and cuddle. I've a couple girlfriends who've told me how horny they were during their pregnancies. What's up with that?"*

You may not be in the mood, and your partner may be afraid to engage in it with you, but the good news is that *vaginal sex* is safe during pregnancy, unless you are having pregnancy-related problems and your health care provider has informed you otherwise (which may be the case if, for instance, there is a concern over preterm labor or if you're having unexplained vaginal bleeding). That also means most sexual positions are safe, so your only limitation may be the discomfort that some positions can cause as your pregnancy progresses.

As with Linda, *you* may have heard that some women feel much more sexual during pregnancy, but that has not been my experience. In fact, the issue I most deal with relating to sex during pregnancy is a definite lack of interest, sometimes for the whole nine months and beyond. If that is decidedly not the case with you, and you're thinking, "I'm as horny as a teenage boy!" I say: *Enjoy these nine months of sex, free from worry over unintended pregnancy!* For most women, sex and intimacy issues may vary with each new trimester.

**In the first trimester**, between the hormonal changes, fatigue, nausea, and fear of miscarriage, sex is not a high priority for most couples, at least not for the pregnant half, but you can assuredly take the fear of sex causing a miscarriage out of the equation.

**Your second trimester** is your best bet for sex because you may be feeling more energetic and have not yet gained too much weight. Chances are you're shopping for the baby, and you're getting along with your partner and generally enjoying the ride.

**The third trimester** may bring around some mild to severe lower back pain, as you are, by now, carrying thirty or more pounds of baby weight. You're feeling swollen all over, including your vagina, and you're losing urine on a daily basis. Due to the increase in blood flow to every organ, the vagina also feels more swollen. Most women notice an engorged feeling in this last trimester, especially during sexual stimulation or intercourse—because of this, the vaginal tissue becomes deeper red or purple in color. Despite assurances to the contrary, you may be worrying that sex will throw you into labor. For all these reasons, sex is not a priority.

That said, I do like to inform my full-term patients that vaginal sex has a great deal of benefit in bringing you to the finish line. Semen contains *prostaglandins*, hormone-like substances that help to ripen, soften, and prepare the cervix for labor and delivery. Joy Sedlock, a certified nurse-midwife from the Cleveland Clinic, says it best when she tells her patients, "What got you in this situation can help get you out!"

Certain questions and concerns regarding sex during pregnancy remain a constant in my own practice. At the top of this list—*and the envelope, please...*

## *Can Sex Harm the Baby?*

The good news is that the baby is surrounded by one to two liters of fluid contained in the amniotic sac (or membranes), which serves as a protective cushion during sex. The baby may bounce, but be assured that she/he is safe and insulated.

### *Are There Better Sexual Positions Than Others?*

Comfort is a priority for the pregnant woman, and finding comfortable positions is important, as many women experience sex differently while they are pregnant. Certain positions involving deeper penetration—such as you, the pregnant partner, on top or in front—may make sex uncomfortable for you. You may also tend to feel nauseous on your back during pregnancy. Sideways positions tend to be the most comfortable. That said, since most sexual positions are perfectly safe, it's up to you and your partner to determine which are the most comfortable and enjoyable.

### *I'm Having a Hard Time, Emotionally, with the Weight Gain.*

Insecurity in one's body image is difficult to anticipate, but, with each visit to your OB, when you're asked to climb aboard that scale, you're reminded about your weight gain. Even if you know that weight gain is right and natural during pregnancy, it can be hard to maintain your pre-pregnant sexual state of mind when you come up against body insecurity. For some women, gaining more than five pounds is emotionally devastating. While your partner may appreciate your enlarged breasts, you may not feel the same appreciation. Weight gain and the body changes it brings are the hardest things for women to overcome, and they may present an obstacle for getting naked in the bedroom.

### *How Common Is Spotting During Vaginal Intercourse?*

Short answer: Very—depending on what trimester you're in. In the first trimester, if you notice spotting with intercourse, it may be due to the implantation of the embryo. Twenty-five percent of women normally have spotting or mild bleeding unrelated to intercourse. If bleeding is in the second or third trimester, the increase blood flow to the cervix may be causing some spotting. Sex with deeper penetration—from behind or with you on top—is also a common cause of spotting. But let's be clear: Spotting is the light blood noticed when you wipe after peeing. It is the kind of blood similar to that first day of your period. Mild or heavier bleeding can be a sign of something more concerning, such as an abnormal implantation of the placenta, called placenta previa. If you have cramping and persistent bleeding, you should contact your health care provider.

### *Are There Any* Real *Reasons Not to Be Sexually Active During Pregnancy?*

Yes, certainly. If you're experiencing any kind of vaginal bleeding or pain with sex, and/or uterine contractions before the thirty-seventh week, if you have been diagnosed with placenta previa, or you have an incompetent cervix, or any other high-risk pregnancy complications, you should speak to your health care provider about any form of sexual intimacy.

### *Vibrators and Sex Toys and Fingers—Oh, My! Are They Safe During Pregnancy?*

Yes, yes, and yes. Vibrators and sex toys are safe, as long as they are washed and cleaned in order to decrease the risk of bacterial or yeast infections. Naturally, the same can be said for fingers inserted into the vagina. Make sure your or your partner's hands are clean—this means fingernails as well.

### *What About Oral Sex?*

Safe. Safe to give and to receive. You've probably heard that your partner should not blow air into your vagina as it can cause an air embolism. Though that is quite rare, it can be a life-threatening condition for you and the baby.

### *Anal Sex?*

Anal sex is generally not recommended during pregnancy because it may introduce bacteria from the rectum into the vagina, which may affect the fetus. However, if you've had anal sex prior to getting pregnant and are accustomed to it, it may be a more comfortable solution to vaginal intercourse. Some partners prefer it to vaginal sex. Be forewarned: if you have hemorrhoids, anal sex will make them all the more bothersome.

And, since we're on the subject of harmful bacteria, remember that STDs (sexually transmitted diseases) are still a possibility with new partners, non-monogamous partners, and partners with STIs (sexually transmitted infections) or unknown STI status, and can present a danger to the fetus. To prevent transmission with such partners, expectant mothers should use condoms.

### *Will I Go Into Labor If I Have an Orgasm?*

When you orgasm, your uterus contracts, but it is not the same type of contraction that occurs in labor. Unless you have signs of *uterine irritability* or *preterm labor*, orgasms during a normal pregnancy will not cause you to go into labor.

### *Is Orgasm Different During Pregnancy?*

Pregnant or not, when you have an orgasm, your muscles tighten and relax. Blood flow increases to the genital area and your uterus contracts rhythmically. When your uterus is normal sized—about the size of a pear—you may not even notice your uterus is contracting. However, when you are, say, twenty weeks pregnant and your uterus is the size of a melon, you are quite aware of that contraction. At forty weeks, when your uterus is the size of a nice, ripe watermelon, you are even more aware of it. The rhythmic contractions you feel as a result of orgasm are short lived and don't persist. It's an old wives' tale that orgasms can force you into labor. It doesn't hurt to try to have an orgasm, with or without your partner—which may be to say that pregnant women sometimes have a low sex drive for sex with their partner and are more interested in masturbation. It's understandable that pregnant women are anxious about causing harm to their baby, or causing preterm labor, but an orgasm will do neither.

Since having an orgasm requires your most important and largest sex organ—your mind—it's important for that mind to be free of worry in order to be in the right mental state to allow an orgasm to happen.

## Generally Speaking, On Sex and the Preggers V…

During pregnancy, a majority of pregnant women prefer the intimacy and closeness of cuddling and kissing with their partners to sexual intercourse. As with any sexual encounter, good communication and respect for emotional and psychological boundaries has to be a priority for you and your partner. One partner may want to have sex more often than the other, who may feel obligated to maintain the pre-pregnancy sexual routine. Discussion of these issues, while respecting each other's concerns, can help bring about some resolution. Maybe vaginal lubrication is all that's needed to make your sexual experience complete. Listen to your body and realize that pregnancy introduces a whole host of new circumstances in the bedroom (and, maybe, other venues).

As I said in the beginning, I do believe a pregnant vagina works in superhero capacity, but that's not to say that it doesn't need its own superhero care. In fact, I believe that mothers should be afforded a one-year body recovery pass after pulling off the super feat of childbirth! Despite all the best preparation in the world, pregnancy—the most challenging hormonal cycle—is alternately overwhelming, terrifying, and blissful, and the changes in your body may be wild and unpredictable, but they're temporary. I encourage all of you mamas-to-be to ask any and every question that occurs to you. Your journey needs to include your partner, your health care provider, and others who may constitute your pregnancy support team. Keep the dialogue continuous, your inquiry boundless, and your attention acute to your body and vagina. If in doubt about any changes or symptoms, do not trust the wisdom of Doctor Google—rather, talk to your doctor. Above all, try to enjoy these nine months, and don't overlook what helped you get here in the first place...hello, vagina!

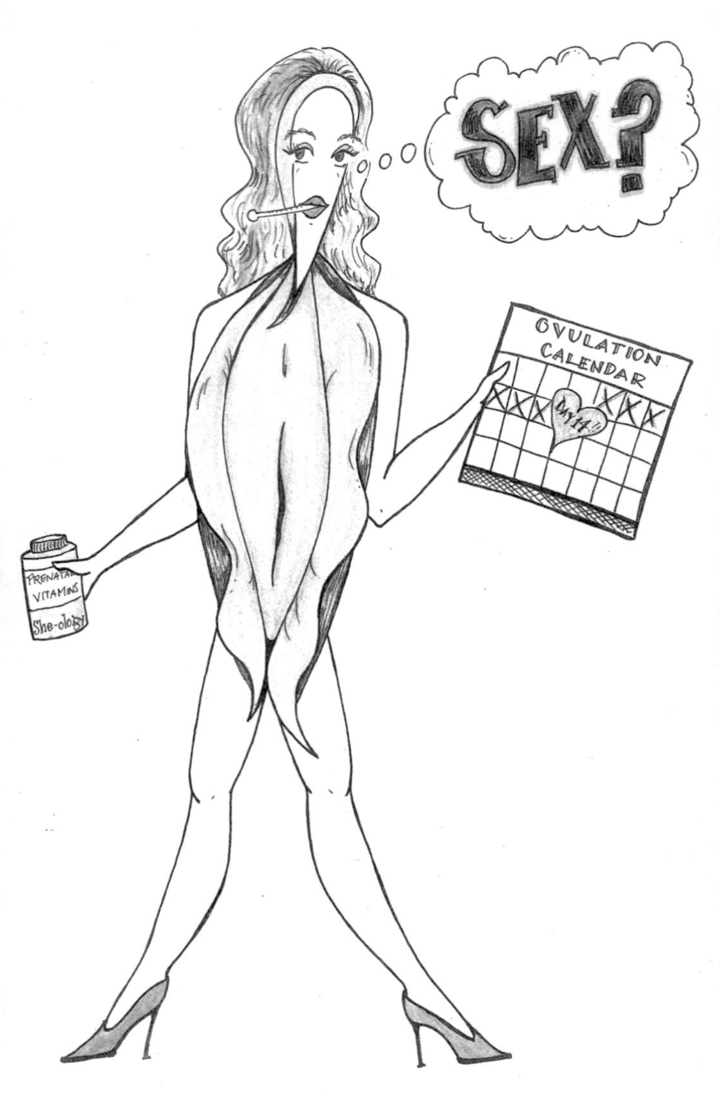
SEX?
OVULATION CALENDAR
Day 14!
PRENATAL VITAMINS
She-ology

CHAPTER 7

# infertile

"Like a lot of women who juggle kids, family, and a career—and maybe take care of an elderly parent as well. Hello?—I'm super busy. I've been the lifestyle and beauty expert on *The Ellen Show* for fifteen years, in addition to taping a daily live segment five days a week on Hallmark's *Home & Family Show*.

Wearing so many hats and wanting to wear them as fabulously as possible, it's not surprising that the thing I managed to neglect was my own self-care. I figured that, if I were vertical and moving, I must be fine. *Finally*, after three years of missed Pap smears, blood tests, colonoscopies, and mammograms, I hired a health concierge service to stay on my back about catching up. Finally, I managed to take care of it all, except the mammogram. For that, I had to find a gynecologist, because I hadn't seen one in *years*.

All the ladies at Hallmark Channel's *Home & Family* show went to Dr. Sherry, so off I went. Dr. Sherry insisted I go for a mammogram

ASAP, so, of course I put it off, again—I was too busy, remember? I pushed it three months, then another three months, and then again, until I was too embarrassed to tell Dr. Sherry I hadn't gone, so I went. Done. Back to busy.

Three days later, I received a call from the radiologist telling me that they saw *something concerning*. He recommended I see my gynecologist for a diagnostic mammogram referral. I ran back to Dr. Sherry, who basically talked me off a ledge and made certain I followed through. She told me that a diagnostic could come back negative. Unfortunately, that wasn't the case. Instead, they wanted to biopsy.

From the biopsy, we found out I had DCIS, ductal carcinoma in situ, which means that the cells lining the milk ducts were cancerous but had not spread into surrounding breast tissue. DCIS is considered non-invasive breast cancer—like, *pre*-Stage I, Stage zero, in fact. In many cases, the cells are in a small, concentrated area, removable by lumpectomy. In my case, the cells were around my entire breast, areola, and nipple. Dr. Sherry insisted I have a mastectomy. In fact, it was her opinion that I have a double mastectomy, just to be sure—the procedure was not something that anyone would want to do *twice*. A double it was—just like the doctor ordered.

And thank God.

The last scoop of breast tissue, which was taken from somewhere nearly hidden *in between* my breasts, revealed cells that were Stage 3 cancer. Had both breasts not been removed, the cancer would have gone undetected and most likely traveled into my lungs. I would probably not be here to write this, if that had been the case.

Which brings me to this plea: Self-care, ladies—please, make it a priority. In addition, find yourself a truly great gynecologist. How do you know if they're great? Well, if they're like Dr. Sherry, they will text you back with critical info, walk you through your worries, and treat you as though you're a valued friend. And they might save your life.

Another thing I would say: You can't be your best, most powerful, and nurturing, warrior self—and we women are nothing, if not warriors—if you're not putting yourself at the top of your list. Be in touch with your body. It is the vehicle for your soul and your psyche and your power. Listen to it as you would listen to someone you love.

With that, with love, Kym. ”

—**Kym Douglas** Television Host, Actress, Author, Fashion and Lifestyle Expert

Once a woman hits puberty she can expect to have about 300,000 to 500,000 eggs in reserve. Now, if you think that's a lot, imagine this: A female fetus at twenty weeks' gestation has about six to seven *million* eggs. By the time that fetus becomes a full-born baby girl, that number drops to between one and two million. So, in answer to a question I often hear from women, "At what age do I start losing eggs?" the answer is: from the time *before* you are born.

By the age of thirty-five, a woman is left with about 25,000 eggs, and, by fifty-one—the typical age of the onset of menopause—the count is down to a thousand. To add insult to injury, the quality of eggs drops at an accelerated pace after the age of forty-two.

As much as I believe in—and live by—the credo that women get better with age, in regard to fertility, aging sucks. However, there are many other factors to understand and take into consideration when discussing the "I" word—infertility—as well as there are steps a woman can take to optimize her chance of avoiding infertility, and options available *if*, indeed, infertility is the cause of an inability to conceive.

So, all that said, let's start with this...

## Are You Really Infertile?

The question of infertility is bandied around these days as the immediate go-to reason as to why, if a woman has been trying to become pregnant, she is unable to conceive. But there are so many variables to take into consideration when deciding on a prognosis as frustrating and heartbreaking as infertility. For instance, what is your general health like? What is the health of your partner like? What is your emotional state of mind, and, most importantly, your *gynecological history*? Also—and this is a big factor—do you have any idea when, in fact, you are *ovulating*?

If you've been trying to become pregnant and it hasn't happened after, say, four months, or five or six, don't panic. Take a step back. For a woman under thirty-five, infertility *may* be the culprit if she is unable to conceive after *twelve* months of actively trying. That means twelve months of unprotected sex *at the right time* (more on this in a bit). However, when taking maternal age and/or other chronic ailments and health conditions into consideration, a woman may be deemed infertile in failing to conceive after only six months of unprotected sex.

And it may come as a surprise, but only 11 percent of women are actually *infertile*. For whatever reason, those women are unable to produce a healthy egg, or their eggs may be unable to travel to the uterus. Thirty-five percent of infertility is caused by this so-called "female factor."

At least, for fairness' sake, another 40–50 percent of infertility is due to a "male factor"—which can be determined by an abnormal semen analysis. When a semen analysis comes back "abnormal," it means that the shape, volume, and/or motility of the sperm are abnormal in that they cannot find or fertilize a woman's egg. The jokes about sperm refusing to ask directions are boundless, but I can tell you it is no laughing matter. The remaining 10 to 20 percent of infertility cases are unexplained, and therefore not identified as having a male or female factor.

Given those frustrating factors for infertility, the good news is that up to 90 percent of infertile couples will be able to get pregnant and deliver a healthy baby. In the majority of cases, once a diagnosis is made, the proper infertility treatment may be determined, resulting in successful pregnancy. Identifying the problem is often half the battle, after which, a plan of creative medical intervention or technology may be the defining factor in making it to a successful pregnancy and the delivery of a healthy baby.

When faced with a couple dealing with infertility, I always suggest having a short-term plan, as well as a long-term plan composed of treatment options and alternatives. It may take longer than imagined to become pregnant, but, with a plan in place, the wait may prove to be a little more bearable.

*Natasha and Tony were a newly married couple in their early thirties, just beaming with health and vitality. In fact, they'd spent a two-week honeymoon camping out in the Yosemite Park before coming to me for a consultation. Apparently, they had been trying to conceive for six straight months, having sex nearly every day—sometimes twice a day—without any luck. I asked Natasha if she was having regular periods—which she was—and if she knew when she was ovulating during the month. Natasha told me she had absolutely no clue as to when her ovulation occurred.*

Unfortunately, Natasha is not alone when it comes to being unaware of one's time of ovulation. Key in terms of becoming pregnant (or, in fact, avoiding pregnancy) is being cognizant of your own menstrual cycle, since good timing for sex is of greater importance than *more* sex. As I told Natasha and Tony, you don't necessarily need to cut back, you just need to be more accurate in your *timing*.

## Understanding the Fertility Window of a Menstrual Cycle or A Brief Biology Lesson on Conception

It is essential to understand when, during your menstrual cycle, you are able to conceive, since it is during the twenty-four-hour period of ovulation that an egg is actually available to be fertilized.

On *average*, women have periods every twenty-eight days. Since that is only an average, most women don't have a perfect twenty-eight-day cycle, so it can be challenging to know when an egg is available for conception. Typically, ovulation occurs fourteen days prior to the start of a period. Some women produce a slimy, egg white-type discharge during ovulation, while others experience twinges or slight pelvic discomfort—some women may experience both discharge *and* discomfort. Whatever your "signs," knowing when your ovulation occurs will make timed intercourse a rather straightforward process—depending on the cooperation and schedule of your partner.

Since sperm lives up to five days inside a woman's body, the idea is to have the sperm *wait* for the egg. For example, if you have determined that you ovulate on Day Fifteen of your cycle—Day One counting as the first day of your period—then your timed intercourse must be on Day Fourteen, Fifteen and

Sixteen. Having intercourse on these days ensures that the sperm and egg are *interfacing*—which is basically the medical term for *rendezvousing*—in the hope of forming an embryo. Additionally, due to the long life cycle of sperm, some experts suggest having intercourse on Day Nine or Ten and then abstaining until Day Fourteen. That way, there is *fresh sperm* ready to find the egg in the fallopian tube, where fertilization takes place.

The best way for you to optimize that fertilization is to keep track of your period cycle, and the best way to do that is through a period tracker—available as an app. Once you've tracked your period for four to six months, you may then bring the information to the attention of your gynecologist so that you may further your fertility conversation in a productive manner.

Not only do my patients love all the amazing period tracker apps now available to them, I can't help but love them as well. When my patients are prepared, it helps me to get right down to the nitty-gritty of their fertility questions. In understanding the timing involved in conceiving, you can understand why it may take an average of six to nine months to become pregnant.

Depending on your age, with timed intercourse, you have a 25 percent chance of conceiving each month. In timing intercourse over a three-month period, 50–60 percent of couples will conceive. Over the course of six months, that percentage jumps to 80 percent. For couples between the ages of twenty and forty-four, 90 percent will conceive after twelve months of timed intercourse. A word here: patience.

However, these statistics refer to couples where there are no red flags. There are, in fact, many factors that can affect fertility—genetics, age, diet, body weight, lifestyle, medical, and contraceptive history and stress.

## Potential Red Flags

The following could signal a difficulty in conceiving:

* **History of Irregular Periods:** Irregular periods can be a potentially serious concern, as it relates to regular ovulation and fertility. Any abnormal (irregular) bleeding patterns may be a sign of underlying health conditions, such as polycystic ovarian syndrome (PCOS), thyroid and prolactin dysfunction, peri-menopause, and premature ovarian failure, all of which can affect your ability to ovulate regularly and conceive naturally.
* **History of Pelvic Inflammatory Disease (PID):** PID can damage the fallopian tubes, which can present serious difficulties when trying to conceive. A history of any sexually transmitted infection, such as Chlamydia and Gonorrhea, can cause tubal disease or tubal scaring which can affect the transport of an egg through the fallopian tube, which is where the fertilization of the egg happens.
* **Two or More Miscarriages in a Row:** Two percent of women will experience two miscarriages in a row, and 1 percent will suffer recurrent miscarriages—two or more in a row. It's fairly well known that the biggest risk factor for miscarriage is age—*older mom* means older and less healthy eggs. Therefore, the older you are when you conceive, the greater the likelihood of miscarriage. The majority of miscarriages (60 percent)

occurs randomly and is due to genetic abnormality, and it's women in their late thirties and early forties that are more likely to miscarry due to those abnormalities. Which leads us back to....

* **Maternal Age:** Women over the age of forty-five have a less than *1 percent* chance of conceiving—even when the timing is right. As significantly as fertility declines in one's mid-thirties, that decline speeds up even more as a woman closes in on forty—amplifying the sound of that proverbial biological clock. Over the age of forty, a woman's eggs are not only less available, but they are of poorer genetic quality. "[A woman's] chance of conceiving at age forty-two is about 9 percent per cycle," explains Dr. Pasquale Patrizio, director of the Yale Fertility Center. By forty-five, a woman trying to conceive will have a greater than 80 percent chance of miscarriage—compared to a 20 percent chance for a woman under thirty. Blood tests can help define the health of a woman's eggs—referred to as her *ovarian reserve*—but there is simply no arguing the facts with regard to biological clocks and fertility, despite how youthful a woman may feel or look.
* **Weight:** Obesity/Underweight can negatively affect fertility. A BMI (body mass index) in the obese range, BMI > 30 percent, increases the risk of infertility due to ovulation problems. Underweight women, BMI < 17 percent, have a low amount of body fat, which may also cause irregular ovulation. And as I've discussed, irregular ovulations can make it a challenge to conceive. Studies have also shown that obesity and extreme thinness can lead to abnormalities in a woman's eggs.

* **Cigarette Smoking:** Not surprisingly, also affects fertility by increasing the chance of miscarriage. Heavy smoking, especially for a long period of time, causes poor egg quality and early menopause. Not only do female smokers need more ovary-stimulating medications during IVF (in vitro fertilization) they wind up with fewer eggs at retrieval time and have a 30 percent lower rate of pregnancy compared with non-smokers that do IVF. Also, because smoking damages the genetic material in eggs and sperm, miscarriage and birth defect rates are higher among patients who smoke. Incidentally, men who were born to mothers who smoked half a pack of cigarettes a day or more had lower sperm counts than men born to non-smokers. Apparently, smoking is the gift that keeps on giving.
* **Endometriosis:** The most common symptoms of endometriosis are related to pain, which can be chronic and disruptive. Pain associated with endometriosis is more commonly seen before and during a period and may include lower back and pelvic pain, and pain during sex. Forty percent of women with infertility suffer from this chronic condition; however, some women don't have any symptoms at all.
* **Uterine Fibroids:** Uterine fibroids are the most common benign pelvic tumors in women. Also known as leiomyomas and myomas, the size and shape of these fibroids vary and can be located anywhere in and around the uterus, negatively affecting a woman's ability to conceive and carry a baby to term.

* **History of Multiple Pelvic Surgeries:** Pelvic surgeries can lead to widespread scarring and damaging of the fallopian tubes, having the same effect as PID. For example, a ruptured appendix can lead to extensive pelvic scarring, making conception impossible.
* **Pituitary Adenomas:** Pituitary adenomas are benign tumors that can secrete excessive amounts of the hormone prolactin, thereby disrupting a woman's period and ovulation. It's common for women with pituitary adenomas to have irregular periods and difficulty conceiving.
* **Medications:** Long-term use of non-steroidal anti-inflammatory drugs (NSAIDs) and aspirin, as well as chemotherapy, radiation, and recreational or illegal drug use (i.e., marijuana or cocaine) can hamper a woman's ability to conceive.
* **Stress:** We know that stress can have a profound effect on one's life. It can cause poor sleep and eating patterns, excessive drinking, drug use, and other unhealthy habits. Stress also leads to depression and anxiety, which can affect fertility; so de-stressing one's life is imperative on the road to pregnancy. In fact, studies show that infertile women who have undergone ten sessions of relaxation training and stress management had *increased* rates of pregnancy (Domar Center at Boston IVF). Along those lines, mindfulness, yoga, and acupressure are commonly used in the process to help reduce stress in order to conceive and have a healthy pregnancy. A psychologist can also be useful in uncovering the causes of stress and anxiety.

While all the aforementioned red flags and deterrents to a healthy pregnancy can seem overwhelming, several of them are issues you may be able take into your own hands. Otherwise, consulting with a health care professional may be your next step in dealing with issues around infertility. Seek out advice and treatment. And, when you seek that advice, go equipped with a list of your concerns and questions. Never feel bad about asking questions. Never.

Now that we've covered what may be standing in your way of conceiving, it's time to look outside of you and to your partner in crime.

## Dude, Is it *You*?

*My patient, Florence, was a thirty-eight-year-old masseuse with a fondness for patchouli. She lived in Castaic, California, with her husband, Paco, a professional weed grower and producer who grew, sold, and smoked A LOT of weed. Every time Florence came to my office, I could tell when her husband was in tow by the intermingling of patchouli and the sweet smell of Paco's artisanal weed. After a year trying to conceive, Florence and Paco were in my office for a consultation.*

If you remember, earlier on, I talked about the "male factor" and how 40–50 percent of infertility is due to that "male factor," which can be determined by a semen analysis (SA). If, indeed, the shape, motility, and volume of your partner's semen are abnormal, it may be that your partner is the cause of your inability to conceive—in which case, it's time for that partner to pay extra special attention to his own personal lifestyle habits. There are many things that can affect a man's sperm count, including:

* Recreational drugs, including marijuana and cocaine
* Medication, including Propecia (Minoxidil), chemotherapy, and radiation therapy
* Varicocele, which is an enlargement of the veins of a man's testicle
* Smoking cigarettes
* Heavy alcohol use
* Pesticides, lead, and other environmental toxins
* Genetic factors
* Obesity
* Stress
* Serious medical conditions, including mumps, kidney, and hormonal abnormalities

Getting a semen analysis is an easy first step to see if your male partner has high-quality sperm and proper motility—that is to say, if your partner is the culprit in your inability to conceive.

* Oh, and one last thing that may affect a man's sperm... age. Does advanced paternal age matter? Yes, it does. Age matters for men—just like it does for women—when it comes to fertility. Not only does a man's age matter when his female partner is trying to conceive, but older sperm has been associated with a higher rate of "psychological disorders and developmental conditions like autism." A JAMA Psychiatry study from 2013 found: "Kids born to men over 45 were 3.5 times more likely to be diagnosed on the autism spectrum and 13 times more likely to be diagnosed with ADHD than those born to the same men when they were 20 to 24."

All that said, if you are thinking about getting pregnant either sometime soon or sometime in the distant future, there are certainly ways to take control of your fertility.

Just as you would train to run a marathon—because pregnancy is nothing if not a marathon—there is a certain amount of mind, spirit, and body training that you can do to ready yourself for the journey. Don't wait for your OB-GYN to initiate a conversation on your fertility. Don't wait for her to ask you whether you're considering pregnancy and what you've done to ready yourself.

In fact, for those of you looking forward to a pregnancy in your near future, I've compiled a list of issues to address before you start to try to conceive. You say you're ready? Okay. On your mark, get set, take time to go through this checklist of preplanning before actually doing the deed. By allowing yourself and your partner the time to do this type of pre-planning, you will be creating the ideal foundation for a healthy pregnancy and, of course, a healthy baby.

## The Preconception Care Check List

1. **Find an OB-GYN.** I know this may seem like a no-brainer, but, before you jump into mapping your ovulation and trying to conceive, find and meet with an OB-GYN—at least six months before you start trying. Speak with your OB-GYN to see if you and your partner are physically and mentally ready to have a healthy pregnancy. If you are, your pregnancy experience will depend significantly on your obstetrician and the hospital she is affiliated with. Find out what your insurance policy covers and interview obstetricians on your plan to make sure you and your

partner are comfortable with the doctor and the hospital. Hospital tours are available and encouraged so you can see firsthand where your baby will be born.

2. **Review your medical history with your doctor.** This is important to ensure that you don't have any underlying medical conditions, such as endometriosis, diabetes, high blood pressure, depression, seizures, or disorders that might cause problems during pregnancy or negatively impact your unborn baby. Proper control of medical conditions *prior* to pregnancy is the key to avoiding problems that can escalate during pregnancy and the post-partum period.
3. **Be aware of your and your family's genetic history.** Genetic or inherited disorders are important to identify prior to conception, since certain disorders can put you and your partner at risk of having a child with an inherited medical condition. If you have a family history of birth defects, diabetes, seizure disorders, and developmental disabilities, that history may impact a child of yours. If you or your partner is Jewish, you would need to have a Tay-Sachs test to see if you are a carrier of the disease, since the disease is typically found in people with certain ancestry, such as Eastern European Jews. Your health care provider can help guide you through pre-existing hurdles.
4. **Have your doctor review all your medication, supplements, herbs, and over-the-counter and prescription medications that you and your partner take on a daily basis.** Even the most seemingly benign of herbs may present a problem in pregnancy—in fact, commonly used herbs such as Dong quai, black cohosh, sassafras, and mugwort are to be avoided pre/during/post pregnancy.

Medications such as Rogaine (Minoxidil), commonly used for hair loss, can also affect the quality of sperm and should *not* be used during the pre-planning period. Antibiotics prescribed for acne, such as Acutane and Tetracycline, also pose potentially harmful side effects to a developing embryo. It's a good idea to avoid aspirin and ibuprofen as well.

5. **Check to make sure that your BMI isn't under 18 or over 30**, as being underweight or overweight can cause hormonal disruptions that can negatively impact ovulation. Maintaining a healthy weight increases your chance of having regular ovulation and affords you a better chance of becoming pregnant.
6. **Substance abuse is one of the leading causes of complications during pregnancy.** Therefore, drug use of any kind, including marijuana, nicotine, alcohol, or other recreational drugs is a no-no. These drugs contain chemicals that are harmful during the pre-planning period and pregnancy by forming byproducts that affect vaginal fluids, quality of sperm, and, ultimately, the ability for an egg and sperm to fertilize. Not only is marijuana known to make sperm hyperactive and less fertile, it's been proven that men who smoke marijuana have a much lower volume of sperm than men who don't partake, and chronic users are found to have cannabinoid in their urine for up to thirty days. In men, tobacco affects fertility by lowering sperm count and causing abnormal-shaped sperm. Women smokers have an increased risk of spontaneous miscarriage and possibly ectopic pregnancy. Pregnant smokers have an increased risk of premature birth, lower birth

weight babies, and sudden infant death syndrome (SIDS). Any and all marijuana and nicotine use should be stopped at least three months prior to attempting pregnancy. Alcohol use should also be stopped, due to its well-known relationship to birth defects. Bottom line: If you and your partner smoke, drink alcohol, or take drugs, it's time to quit and start becoming your healthiest self.

7. **Coffee drinkers, I'm not coming after you.** Rather, there is a safe way to keep up your habit, if you so desire. Initially, moderate caffeine consumption—meaning about 200mg/day, or a twelve-ounce cup of brewed coffee—was thought to be a contributing factor in miscarriages and preterm labor. However, the good, new news for coffee drinkers is that studies currently do not show that moderate caffeine consumption affects your chance of conceiving or leads to an increased miscarriage rate. Relief, right? But it is recommended that you limit your daily caffeine intake to one cup of coffee or two cups of tea during the pre-pregnancy period. Be sure you know how much caffeine is contained in other beverages—and foods—you consume, so that you can keep your consumption under the recommended amount.

8. **STIs.** Because a history of recurrent STIs (sexually transmitted infections) can cause infertility, it is so important to discuss your history with your doctor. Pelvic Inflammatory Disease "PID" is a common pelvic disease caused by STIs, as is Gonorrhea, Chlamydia, and Syphilis. Any of these infections can cause serious and potentially long-term reproductive problems. No matter your history, being tested for STIs should be a part of your checklist.

9. **Vitamins.** Prenatal vitamins are your friends, the most vital of which is folic acid—shown to reduce the chances of spinal defects—which you need to start taking three to six months before conception. Make sure your prenatal or multivitamin contains at least 400mcg to 1mg of folic acid. Additionally, omega-3 fish oil helps with the healthy development of the fetal brain and visual system. It also would be a good idea to find out if you are deficient in any vitamins such as D or B. Fertile One PC 600 is my go-to preconception vitamin, since it has all the essential vitamins and minerals necessary in preparation for pregnancy.
10. **A word about autism and prenatal vitamins:** It stands that about 1.5 percent of eight-year-old boys are "on the spectrum." Although there is a strong genetic component to that statistic, there are also environmental triggers that increase the risk of autism. New studies show a 30 percent decrease risk in autism for babies born to women who took prenatal vitamins with folic acid around the time of conception. Since 50 percent of pregnancies are *unplanned,* and most women do not start taking prenatal vitamins with folic acid unless they are planning to conceive, that means that half the women that conceive do not have the benefit of having taken folic acid *before* becoming pregnant. Given this startling realization, it is recommended that *all women of childbearing age* should be taking a prenatal vitamin to help reduce their risk of having a child born with autism.
11. **Become your healthiest self now.** Use the prospect of pregnancy as an excuse, if need be. If you're not already

doing so, you should be eating a complete and well-balanced whole food, plant-based diet in order to optimize your health and energy level. The Mediterranean diet is a good place to start—and has been embraced by the medical community as a model of healthy living. This style of eating combines a well-balanced diet—focusing on plant-based foods, including fresh fruit, whole grains, along with fish, lean meats, unprocessed foods, and healthy fats—consumed in a relaxed environment. Regular exercise—as little as 30 minutes of moderately intense exercise a day, three to five times a week—will also improve your health and well-being. Exercise can reduce blood pressure, reduce blood sugar levels, lower cholesterol levels, control body weight and body fat, and improve your overall quality of life. Exercise can also help you sleep, and there is nothing more valuable than a good night's rest. Women need an average of six to eight hours of sleep per night. And don't forget to drink...water! Water is vital for every system in our bodies. You need to drink at least eight glasses of water a day for optimal health. Eating well, exercising regularly, and getting a good night's sleep will contribute to your being your healthiest self in preparation for pregnancy, and in preparation for life!

12. **CoQ10 is one of those supplements that may help your fertility.** When taken before conceiving—300 to 600mg a day—it's thought that it might improve the function of eggs by helping their mitochondria produce energy, thereby helping the fertilization process. Once pregnant, you should stop taking CoQ10, since its effect during pregnancy is not well studied.

13. **Avoid vacationing in countries with high Zika exposure.** The Zika virus—which can cause infants to be born with microcephaly and other congenital malformations—is spread to humans primarily from the bite of infected mosquitoes. Humans then pass it to each other primarily through sex. For couples trying to conceive, it is imperative to avoid traveling to states and countries where the Zika virus has been found, at least six months prior to conceiving. The current recommendation is, if your male partner has traveled to an area high risk for Zika, he needs to wear a condom for six months, just to be on the safe side. Use the CDC website to find out the latest locations of the Zika virus. (https://www.cdc.gov/zika/geo/index.html)

Preparation for pregnancy should be thoughtful and deliberate. If you follow the Preconception Care Check List, this will ensure that you are as healthy and well educated as you can be *before* you begin the pregnancy cycle.

But what if you are far away from pursuing pregnancy, either because you feel you are too young to start thinking about kids, or you haven't found the right partner, or you're waiting for your career to fall together first? What if you're not even sure that you may want kids, but you don't necessarily want to close the door on that option *and* you happen to be barreling through your thirties? If anything I've mentioned rings true, then you may want to start thinking about freezing your eggs.

## Freezing Your Eggs... When, How, What?

It seems to me that women of childbearing age have become obsessed about their future fertility, and I think it's actually a good thing! In my personal practice, I have noticed that more and more women in their twenties are asking me about egg freezing as a means of planning for the future.

It used to be that *family planning* meant the use of birth control in order to *prevent* pregnancy, but now egg freezing has given that plan a whole new meaning. Today, better techniques and higher rates of success for freezing eggs have changed the way that women chart their family planning.

A recent study found that the most common reason for a woman to freeze her eggs was a "lack of a current partner, and not only to pursue career advancement." The Guttmacher Institute, a prominent reproductive health think tank, has stated, "controlling family timing and size can be a key to unlocking opportunities for economic success, education, and equality for women." They also found that the choice to freeze one's eggs and therefore delay childbirth "will help increase women's earning power" and ultimately "narrow the gender pay gap." That seems to be a whole lot of valid and encouraging reasoning economically, politically, and socially to choose egg freezing. So the question remains: When do you start to consider that option?

Around your early thirties is the time to have a heart-to-heart with *yourself* and ask the following questions: How many children do I want? Am I willing to get pregnant without having a partner? How important is it to have my own biological child? You don't want to look back when it's too late and say to yourself: I wish I had been proactive in planning for my family.

It's during your early thirties that you may need to bring up the subject of egg freezing to your gynecologist. Don't wait for a general practitioner to offer to help you in your future family planning, as they're often too busy or not in the know for such a specialized conversation. Find a gynecologist and talk to her about whether you're a good candidate for egg freezing.

The best candidates for such a procedure are women between the ages of thirty-one and thirty-eight who are delaying pregnancy by at least two years. For this age group, the success rate of a live birth with either frozen eggs or frozen embryos is 40 to 50 percent.

If you are a healthy woman older than thirty-eight, you need to decide now whether you will freeze your eggs, and then you need to make an appointment with a fertility specialist tomorrow. Women older than forty may be candidates for freezing, but their success rates for pregnancy are less than 10 percent, and the cost may not be worth the odds.

The cost of egg freezing often separates those who can only *think* about the process versus those who can actually *afford* to do it. One cycle of egg freezing can cost around ten thousand dollars, and, often, two cycles are needed to produce a healthy egg account. Fortunately, companies like Facebook and Apple are at the forefront of embracing and protecting a woman's choice to delay motherhood. They are championing their career-driven women employees by supporting them in the family-planning department, which translates into including such support in health insurance benefits.

If you are interested in learning more about egg freezing it's important to meet with an infertility specialist who can walk you through the process. In that process, fertility medications are taken during the first half of your menstrual cycle to hyper-stimulate the ovaries in order to create as many eggs as possible. During this time, you will be closely monitored to make sure you are tolerating the medications well and not experiencing side effects, such as headaches, mood swings, abdominal pain, bloating, and hot flashes. Once your ovaries are primed to create mature and healthy eggs, a vaginal ultrasound with an attached needle is used to reach the ovaries and follicles through the back of the vagina. The fluid inside each follicle contains an egg, which is then aspirated through the needle and suctioned into a sterile container. The eggs retrieved are than stored in a freezer for future use.

Based on the latest findings by The American College of Obstetricians and Gynecologists, which reports that a woman's ability to have babies decreases gradually but significantly beginning around age thirty-two and then goes down more rapidly after age thirty-seven, your early thirties is the prime time to be discussing egg freezing. Don't put yourself in the position of getting too close to the fertility cliff.

There are so many ways in which to be proactive about family planning, ways in which to take control of your life, recognize potential obstacles to becoming pregnant, repair your health, and boost your fertility. The key is to become proactive, because nobody knows better than you whether children are on your mind—be it in the forefront or deep in the recesses of possibility. Stay connected with yourself and your near or distant plans for your future, especially if that future includes a family.

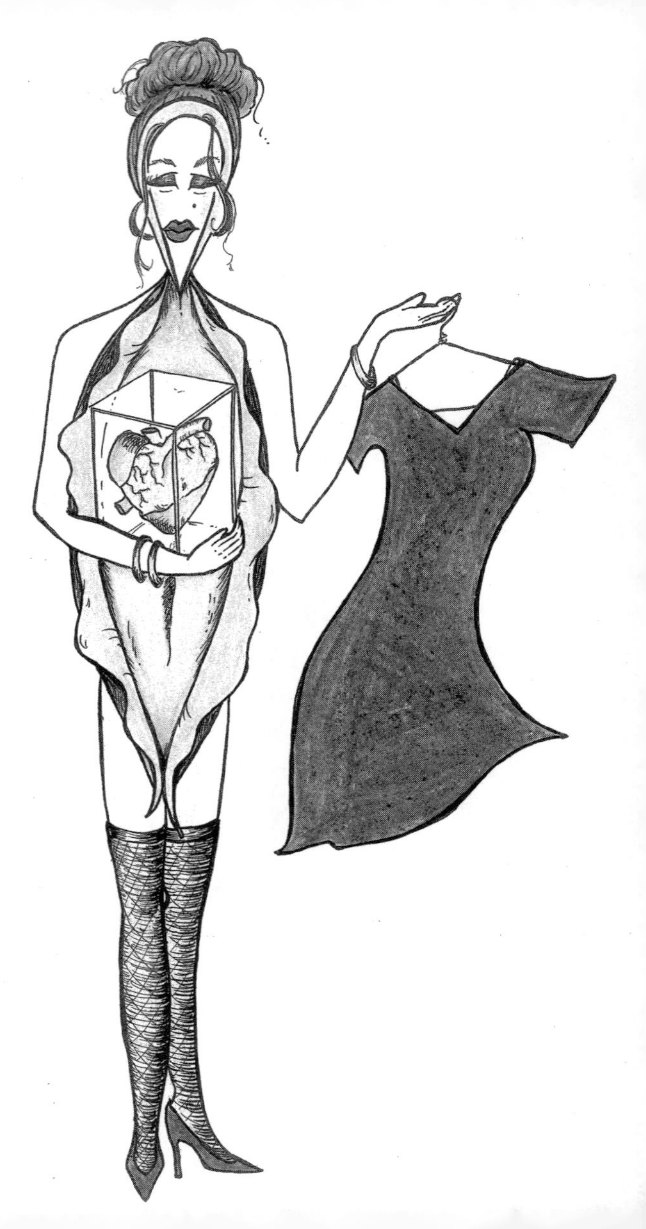

CHAPTER 8

# hearty

"When I was ten, my father died of a 'stroke.' I was too young to know what that meant. Somewhere along the way, in the days after his death—maybe it was over the mashed potatoes and collard greens at the reception—someone explained to me that he had died because there wasn't enough blood to his brain. For a long time, I imagined he had died because there had been something wrong inside his head, inside his brain that seemed so agile with easy jokes, charm for days, and an infectious laugh. As I got older, I learned otherwise, but I only learned half the story about heart disease.

Since movies and pop culture always seemed to reference heart attacks as something that happen to men—it's always the man that grabs his chest and falls to the ground—I'd never thought of heart disease in terms of something that affected women and certainly no one talked about it, over collard greens or otherwise.

Around the time I turned fifty, Dr. Sherry—knowing my family history—suggested I have a stress echocardiogram (SEC), just to have a baseline measure of how well my heart was functioning. I showed up to the cardiologist's office in my compression pants, sports bra, and running shoes, since I knew I'd be running a treadmill. As a long-distance runner, I was excited to test my endurance, a little cocky even. The ego kept saying, 'You're gonna CRUSH THIS TEST.' Before the big 'race,' I had to take off my Nike shirt and super-duper race elite sports bra, to have electrodes pasted to my body, which were connected to wires that protruded from a machine, like tentacles from the Kraken. The med tech had me lie down on an exam table, did an ultrasound of my heart at rest, and then told me to hop on the treadmill. 'Sure,' I said, 'Just let me put my sports bra back on.'

She said, 'Oh, no, it's not compatible with the test to wear a bra.' My heart started racing. Run, with no bra? I said, 'I think it must be illegal in like six states to make a woman run without a bra.' She repeated she was sorry but 'that's just the way it is.'

I flap jacked my way through the stress part of the test. Everything checked out, but, after I left I was hit with the realization of how heart disease had been institutionalized for so long as being very much a man's disease, and how even the test seemed geared towards a man. No one had even imagined what it would be for a woman to perform the test topless, how it would not only affect her ability to run, but her state of mind and well-being in the process. I thought of how many women have been sexually assaulted, of what if the med tech were a man, would someone not go through the test because of a past experience? What would that mean if they were not diagnosed? If she was lucky, how did a woman even find her way to this test? So many questions tumbled in my mind, one over the other.

I did some research and learned that heart disease is the number one killer of women. Number One. A little more research led me to learn that more women die of heart disease than all cancers combined. Statistically speaking, even if you have breast cancer, you're still more likely to die of heart disease. It shocked me to think that I'd gone so long without that information. I invited Dr. Sherry to work with me to improve the stress echocardiogram experience for women and asked her how I could be of service in getting the message out to women regarding heart disease. Dr. Sherry introduced me to the American Heart Association to try to amplify their messaging and we got to work imagining a new SEC experience for women.

As I approach the age my father was when he died, I become more determined in my search to improve the stress echocardiogram and to get the message out to women to pay attention to their bodies and to the information available to them regarding heart disease, to make healthy choices, to exercise. As of this date, Dr. Sherry and I have patented a device that not only makes the SEC experience better for women, but it also improves the accuracy of the test. If I can help prevent another woman from being a heart disease statistic, I'll feel like I've accomplished something worthwhile. ”

—**Jennifer Beals** Actress

As an OB-GYN, I'm not only on the front lines advocating conversations about gynecological health—although *Viva la V!* will always remain my war cry—I'm a health care provider responsible for the *whole* well-being of my female patients. In line with attention to health issues specific to women, I'm greatly concerned about women's *heart health.* The fact is that many women rely on their OB-GYN as their primary health care providers, from the time of first menses to menopause and beyond, so it's imperative to consider that other, equally important lady part: the heart. Your yearly OB-GYN visit—and you are seeing your OB-GYN at least once a year, *right*?—is not only a time to check the plumbing, so to speak, but it's important as a means to learning your personal risk factors of heart disease, and to take the necessary steps in avoiding that particular and uncompromising *heartache*.

Not your worry, you say?

So, if I were to ask you what the most common cause of death among women is in today's society, what would you answer? Auto accidents? Ovarian cancer? Lung cancer? Breast cancer? Predictably, most women answer breast cancer, because the subject of breast cancer and the statistics and treatment options about the disease are so prevalent in women's health books and articles—and rightly so. One in eight women will develop breast cancer in their lifetime. So, if you answered breast cancer, you would be...wrong.

Heart disease, once thought to be primarily a "man's disease," is the number one killer of women. The alarming fact is that one in three women will die of some type of cardiovascular disease, which includes heart disease and stroke. In fact, heart disease accounts for more deaths than all forms of female cancer combined—including breast, lung, and ovarian. The ugly truth of heart disease remains:

* Every eighty seconds a woman dies of cardiovascular disease or stroke.
* An estimated 43 million women in US are affected by heart disease.
* Ninety percent of women have one or more risk factors.
* Fewer women than men survive heart attacks, primarily because the symptoms not only can be different

in women than in men, those symptoms are often misunderstood!

* Only 17 percent of women consider heart disease or stroke to be the greatest health problem facing Americans today.

However, there is a ray of light in these distressing facts and figures: 80 percent of heart disease can be prevented! This promising statistic has put me on a mission to raise awareness among women as to how they may be proactive in recognizing risk factors and preventing heart disease in the first place!

*Karen is one of those women who takes advantage of any time and place to grab a moment of exercise—that includes bounding down the hallway of my practice en route to the exam room. Her daily hour-long workouts include cardio, Pilates, Soul Cycle—you name it—so it's no wonder that she is in amazing shape and boasts only 10 percent body fat. That she is vegan, doesn't drink alcohol, and has never touched a cigarette in her life, just about qualifies her for sainthood in my book. Sadly, though, heart disease has taken its toll in Karen's life. Her grandmother died at fifty-three from a heart attack and her mother suffered the same fate at sixty-five. As an African-American woman, Karen is aware that heart disease disproportionately affects black women—7.6 percent of black women, as opposed to 5.8 percent of white women, have heart disease. Suffice to say, Karen is petrified of suffering the same fate as her mother and grandmother, especially since she's just celebrated her fiftieth birthday.*

Standard medical screening protocol for women goes—or should go—something like this: yearly Pap smear, starting at twenty-one in order to check for cervical cancer, mammograms beginning at forty to screen for breast cancer, colonoscopies added at fifty in order to check for colon cancer, along with bone density tests to detect osteoporosis. Heart disease? It affects a third of all women, and, unbelievable as it may seem, there are still no set guidelines for screening.

Somewhere between a patient and those frightening statistics, there must be a health care provider who knows how to fill in the gap with good detective work. So, although there is no one *set screening,* as for breast and cervical cancer, there are yearly tests your health care provider can prescribe for conditions that put women at risk for heart disease and heart attack.

Heart attack. It's a word that, like the word "cancer," can conjure up many conflicting and sometimes false conceptions. In fact, a heart attack can "look" more like a slow ambush than an abrupt strike. For that reason, it's important to know the variables.

## What Is a Heart Attack?

A heart attack occurs when blood flow in the coronary arteries—those arteries that deliver oxygen to the heart—is reduced, limited, or completely restricted. The arteries may be narrowed over time due to high cholesterol, high blood pressure, or diabetes, thus compromising blood flow to the heart—resulting in the oxygen starvation that leads to what's commonly known as a heart attack (or myocardial infarction). Often, there are no warning signs because, when one artery narrows, nearby arteries and blood vessels may expand to compensate for the damaged one.

Just as you've probably seen on *Grey's Anatomy*, the classic symptoms of a heart attack—almost always suffered by a man—include sudden chest pain, cold sweats, and shortness of breath, followed by the man clutching at his chest and crumpling to the floor. However, a silent heart attack, which affects both genders, can present with less specific signs, including flu-like symptoms such as lightheadedness, nausea, vomiting, sweating, severe fatigue, indigestion, jaw or upper back or arm pain (especially in your left arm). It's these types of less specific signs that are more common in women.

Oftentimes, women present with pain, pressure, or discomfort in the chest, which may or may not be severe or seem significant. In fact, the pain may come and go, leading one to believe that since it isn't constant, it's nothing to worry about.

The question remains: How do you know if you already have heart disease or if you're at risk for it?

## Testing for Heart Disease

More than likely, you have your blood pressure taken whenever you go for a visit with your health care provider. That simple test can be the first determinant as to whether you may be at risk for heart disease, but it's only one test. Don't be afraid to ask your health care provider about tests for cholesterol levels as well as fasting glucose or A1C tests, as those screen for diabetes and pre-diabetic conditions. If you've been prescribed these tests already, find out how often you need to be re-checked. Whoever prescribes your screening—your gynecologist or general practitioner—it's as important for you, as it is for them, to be aware of your personal risk factors in order for you to be your own best health advocate.

In addition, if any of these tests show early warning signals of heart disease, there are more advanced diagnostic tests that your health care provider may (and should) insist upon. Those tests include:

* **Electrocardiogram (ECG).** An ECG records electrical signals from the heart, showing its rhythm and structure. An ECG can be done while you are at rest or while exercising.
* **Exercise stress test.** This test monitors how your heart pumps while exercising in order to observe its ability to function while "stressed."
* **Echocardiogram.** An echocardiogram employs ultrasound to view the heart's structure and how well it functions.
* **Holter monitor.** Or simply, Holter. This is a type of electrocardiography device that monitors ECG heart activity over a period of twenty-four to forty-eight hours or longer, if necessary.
* **Cardiac catheterization with X-ray images.** This diagnostic test uses a thin sheath, which is inserted in a groin artery traveling into the heart in order to detect how well the heart is pumping blood.
* **Cardiac Computerized Tomography (CT) scan** or **Cardiac Magnetic Resonance Imaging (MRI).** These are high-tech tools used to evaluate how well the heart is working—one of the differences being that the CT scan involves radiation from X-rays and the Cardiac MRI is radiation free.

In addition to these tests—and sometimes even before any of these tests are done—your health care provider will ask about your personal and family history. It's important to be as honest and concise in your answers as possible. Did your mother's father succumb to a heart attack at age fifty? Have you been experiencing shortness of breath? Are you experiencing excessive swelling in your feet and ankles? Have you recently stopped taking any prescribed medication? Does your current physician know about *all* the prescription medicine you might be taking?

Remember, all these factors may come into play, so, along with being aware of changes in your physical well-being and medication intake, be prepared with a little family research.

## Traditional Risk Factors

As with a family history of cardiovascular disease, there are other certain risk factors. Most of them—and the ones you may already know about—are the same for women as they are for men. Those include:

* **High blood pressure.** This condition means that the force of blood against your artery walls is consistently high enough to put you at risk of heart disease or stroke. Normal blood pressure has a systolic number (referring to the upper number) of less than 120 and a diastolic (lower number) of less than 80. A systolic and diastolic reading of greater than 130/80 is considered high blood pressure, and, quite dramatically, a "silent killer," as high blood pressure does not usually have symptoms. You won't know you have high blood pressure unless you're *tested*.

* **High Lipid Panel.** This refers to one's cholesterol level. A high lipid panel suggests that the "bad" cholesterol is accumulating in the inner walls of arteries, narrowing them and causing them to become atherosclerotic, which means narrow and hardened. Blood clots can then form, blocking and narrowing arties, increasing your risk of a heart attack or stroke.
* **BMI>30 (BMI greater than 30).** BMI is the measure of body fat, based on one's height and weight. A normal BMI is considered to be 18.5 to <25, overweight is 25–29.9 BMI.
* **Tobacco Use.** Cigarette smoking causes 30 percent of all heart disease deaths. Need I say more?
* **Genetic influences.** Yes, unfortunately, your family history of heart disease can put you at risk.
* **Physical Inactivity.** The findings are everywhere. Physical inactivity puts you at a major risk for cardiovascular disease. Get up and move!

As I mentioned, all of the aforementioned risk factors are the same in women as they are in men. But, as Dr. Nanette Wenger, a leading cardiologist in women and heart disease suggests, "[since] a woman is not a small man, when assessing the cardiovascular risks for women, we need to look beyond traditional risk factors by examining the *natural hormonal cycles* unique to women." Those particular factors include:

* **Pregnancy Complications**
* **Oral Contraception**
* **Hormonal Infertility Therapy**
* **Hormone Replacement Therapy (HRT)**

And, although the following are not unique to women, they seem to pose a greater risk factor—perhaps by their predominance—in women:

* **Systemic Autoimmune Diseases such as Rheumatoid Arthritis, Lupus, and Psoriasis**
* **Depression**

It can certainly be argued that, if men were the ones who gave birth, there would be a lot less pregnancies—as Gloria Steinem said: "If men could get pregnant, abortion would be a sacrament"—but, until then, due to pregnancy, birth, and hormones, women unfortunately face greater risk of cardiovascular problems than men.

## Risks for Women (Facts and Myths)

*Roxanne is a healthy forty-five-year-old mother of IVF twin eight-year-old girls, but her road to pregnancy was a fierce physical and emotional battle. After she and her husband spent six years and all their energy on a business for building sustainable homes for families of color, they were finally ready to start a family of their own. Five years and five miscarriages (one at six months) later, they were able to get pregnant using donor eggs. Roxanne's pregnancy was spent mostly in bed with severe morning sickness, resulting in a five-pound weight loss by twelve weeks, followed by preterm labor at twenty-eight weeks, high blood pressure at thirty-four weeks, and a C-section at thirty-six weeks—fortunately for Roxanne, she had a husband by her side who massaged her aching back for hours on end and serenaded her on guitar. Eight months after the successful delivery of her twin girls, Roxanne's high blood pressure remained difficult to treat. At thirty-eight, she scheduled her first cardiologist appointment for heart disease screening.*

### *Pregnancy*

One of the first great stress tests that can often predict a woman's future health is pregnancy—arguably one of the most joyful hormonal cycles. Pregnancy complications such as hypertension of pregnancy (known as preeclampsia), preterm labor, and gestational diabetes can reveal early predictions for cardiovascular risk and uncover vulnerabilities in various organs. That is to say, the effects of pregnancy can last for far longer than the actual pregnancy and postpartum period!

If a woman experiences some form of disease of the blood vessels—especially preeclampsia or gestational diabetes—during her pregnancy, once that pregnancy is over, those complications and concerns can persist. For instance, if a woman experiences preeclampsia, her chance of having hypertension later in life increases three- to sixfold, and her risk of heart disease and stroke is twice as great as that of a woman who had an uneventful pregnancy. Women who suffer gestational diabetes are seven times as likely to become diabetic. And it's not only *later* in life—meaning menopause and beyond—that the results of these pregnancy complications can be felt; they can occur several years after pregnancy, while a woman is *still* in her childbearing years.

Therefore, in order to reduce the risks of cardiovascular disease later in life, it's important to follow up with a cardiologist for the appropriate testing. A detailed pregnancy history is also key to assessing those risks. Seriously, don't wait until those later years to assess your cardiovascular health. Don't assume that because you are still of childbearing age that you're exempt from the blood diseases associated with "older" folks. Cardio disease is definitely nonpartisan when it comes to age.

## *Oral Contraception (OCP) and Heart Disease: Is There a Connection?*

It has been an ongoing argument: whether or not oral contraception contributes to the risk of heart disease. So, in light of the fact that 23 percent of reproductive age women in the United States use oral contraception, I'd like to put that argument to rest. There is *no* increased risk of heart disease in a *healthy* woman that has *no risk factors* to begin with. However, if you use OCP and *smoke cigarettes* you do have a sevenfold increased risk of heart disease. So let's be clear: You should not be on OCP if you smoke, especially if you are over the age of thirty-five; also, if you have hypertension, you do have a small increased risk of stroke.

In effect, if you have known coronary risk factors such as hypertension, or you're a cigarette smoker, you should seek advice from your health care provider or OB-GYN as to whether or not the coronary risk outweighs the pregnancy risk. And don't despair if OCP isn't for you. Healthy birth control options are available. The IUD and diaphragm are great alternative methods and come with negligible or no risk.

## *Hormonal Infertility Therapy and Heart Disease*

If you're undergoing or have undergone hormonal infertility treatment, don't rush to any hand wringing, but it now seems that there may be a new risk factor for heart disease in women with a history of infertility hormonal treatment. Now, here's the rub: It seems that a large study conducted in Canada from 1993 to 2010 showed that the new risk factor applies to women with *unsuccessful* fertility treatment. However, women who had *successful* fertility therapy had a *decrease* in the number of deaths due to stroke, mini-stroke (TIA), thromboembolism, and heart failure compared to the general population.

The findings from this study might, not surprisingly, stress out women who have undergone failed infertility treatments, but there are other factors to keep in mind. This study does not necessarily mean that if you had unsuccessful fertility treatments you are, without a doubt, at increased risk. Rather, the findings state a "correlation, not a causation." The risk of heart disease for those women who didn't have successful infertility treatment is present, but it is very low. The findings may also mean that those women already had "pre-existing heart conditions or a predisposition to heart disease that [were] discovered or unmasked through fertility treatments," said Dr. Janet Choi, a reproductive endocrinologist who heads CCRM-New York, one of the nation's leading fertility treatment centers. She added, "Women who are infertile tend to be older and have potentially undiagnosed medical issues which could increase their risk for later life cardiovascular events." As for the study, it's quite possible that medical history—including relatively advanced age (for childbearing) obesity, high cholesterol, and blood pressure, and smoking—may not have been taken into consideration.

The most important takeaway from this study is that women need to share every aspect of their medical history with their health care providers, especially if they have a history of failed infertility treatment. Whether or not you've been put at increased risk for heart disease is not completely clear, but it should be considered when addressing your risk factors.

## *Menopause, Hormone Replacement Therapy (HRT), and Heart Disease*

Ah, yes, menopause—that great hormonal cycle game changer and subject of varying and ongoing conversations regarding heart disease.

Prior to going into menopause, the hormone estrogen has a positive and healthy effect on blood vessels and blood flow, but, once you enter menopause, estrogen levels plummet and the experience is typically one of hormonal chaos, resulting in emotional and physical upheaval.

The decrease in estrogen levels during menopause *may* increase risk of heart disease but does not *cause* cardiovascular disease. Although it is not recommended as a treatment for cardiovascular disease, hormone replacement therapy (HRT) can be used to safely treat other disruptive symptoms of menopause, including hot flashes, night sweats, insomnia, and mood changes.

If you're dealing with menopause—and it's almost like a career in itself for many of us—increases in blood pressure, LDL (the bad cholesterol) and triglyceride levels may be expected—my best advice is to concentrate on all-around healthy habits instead of worrying about possible added risks. If you aren't already making changes to your diet and lifestyle for the better, menopause should be your wake-up call.

### *Systemic Autoimmune Diseases, Depression, and Heart Disease*

If you have a health care provider who's on the ball, and you suffer from systemic autoimmune diseases, including rheumatoid arthritis, Lupus, and Psoriasis, you may already know that you are at an increased risk of heart disease. If you haven't had a conversation about your risks due to these common medical conditions, it's time, even if you feel you're too young to worry. The earlier you realize your risks, the better the chance at beating the odds. Discuss your risk with your health care providers to set up early screening and preventative management.

Also, it may come as no surprise that depression is also an elevated risk factor in heart disease, as are high-risk behaviors that include drug use and cigarette smoking. If you suffer from depression, if you're still smoking, or you're relying on certain prescribed or recreational drugs, realize the effect it has on your heart system and take the steps necessary to help yourself move forward with health and an open heart.

### *Heart Disease and Ethnicity*

The American Heart Association reports that only 17 percent of women consider heart disease or stroke to be the greatest health problem facing Americans today. Even more worrisome is that African-American women are the least likely among *all* women to consider heart disease or stroke as the greatest health problem facing them. In fact, only 13 percent consider it so, and that number is nearly as great in Hispanic and Asian women.

This is especially distressing because nearly half of African-American women and a third of Hispanic women suffer from heart disease. In my opinion, the medical community is simply not doing an effective job at getting the message of this elevated risk out to women of color. Nor are health care providers *providing* the necessary information on how to be proactive in the fight against heart disease.

Women of all ages and skin color need to be made aware of their risks in order to take immediate action.

### *Pesticides, Metal Exposure, and Heart Disease*

Recent studies show a connection between an increased risk of heart disease and high blood pressure and ongoing exposure to pesticides, solvents, and metals. Researchers at the University of Illinois at Chicago discovered that workers exposed to pesticides were 2.2 times more likely to suffer coronary heart disease, six times more likely to have heart arrhythmias, and had a 38 percent higher risk of blood vessel damage in the brain than workers without such exposure.

Women at risk for heart disease may want to think twice about working in environments that further increase their risk. However, if you don't have a choice, there are steps you can take to minimize your workplace exposure, such as working in a well-ventilated space, using protective equipment such as gloves, eyewear, or respirators, and washing the part of your body that comes in contact with hazardous materials.

## Healthy Heart Habits

Whether you are twenty-five or sixty-five, you are never too young or too old to form healthy habits. Of course, it's better to start earlier, but you can take hold of control at any age. Understand your family's medical history as well as your own.

Look at your health and understand the changes that may need to be made in your daily choices and in your lifestyle.

As early as your twenties—and at whatever age you may be right now—the following are ways to grab hold of a healthier way of living:

1. **Eat a healthy diet.** Yes, period. If you've made a promise to yourself (or a loved one) to follow such a diet, and you continually *cheat,* you're only cheating yourself. A diet focused on fresh fruits, vegetables, whole grains, and fish, limited alcohol intake, and little red meat (similar to the Mediterranean diet) shows health benefits that include:

   * Reduced risk of cardiovascular disease and stroke
   * Lowered risk of Type 2 Diabetes
   * Reduced risk of a stroke
   * Improved cognitive function
   * Slowed progression of carotid plaque—the fatty deposits that clog blood vessels
   * Cardiovascular *protection.* A Mediterranean diet has been shown to lower total carotid plaque, LDL cholesterol, HDL cholesterol, triglycerides, blood pressure, and blood sugar.

     Along with the Mediterranean diet, the Dietary Approaches to Stop Hypertension (DASH) diet and the Ornish diet are associated with the highest life expectancy and lowest heart disease rates in the world.

     The DASH diet—which is promoted by the National Heart, Lung and Blood Institute—emphasizes much the same foods as the Mediterranean diet, such as fruits, veggies, whole grains, lean protein, and low-fat dairy. It discourages foods high in sodium, saturated fat, and sugar. In fact, it tied with U.S. News' Best Overall Diet rankings at number one.

In that same ranking, the Ornish diet—created by Dr. Dean Ornish, a clinical professor of medicine—not only encourages a diet low in fat, refined carbs, and animal protein; it also focuses on the importance of exercise and stress management. Aerobic activity and weight training are as much an emphasis as is good eating, meditation, and healthy relationships!

2. **Avoid certain foods.** Those foods include:
   * **Foods high in saturated fats and trans fats (a.k.a. partially hydrogenated or hydrogenated fats).** We're talking red meat, full-fat dairy products, coconut and palm oils, deep-fried fast food, bakery products, packaged snack foods, margarines, crackers, chips, and cookies.
   * **Foods high in excessive sodium.** As with the DASH diet, it's recommended that you not consume more than 1,500mg/day (.75 tsp) of sodium. Check those labels.
   * **Sugar.** Sugar-sweetened beverages, sweets, grain-based dessert, and bakery foods. Sugar, sugar, sugar, period.
   * **Processed meats.** Sorry, this means no bacon, sausage, hot dogs, pepperoni, salami, and processed deli meats.

3. **Exercise regularly.** This means incorporating some kind of moderate-intensity aerobic activity into your life, ideally, on a daily basis. In fact, new federal exercise guidelines recommend 150 minutes a week of such activity *and* at least two days a week of muscle-strengthening activity.

Brisk walking, jogging, and running are all excellent ways to lower your risk of heart disease. A study at the Cleveland Clinic showed that only 34 percent of Americans were aware of this exercise benchmark, with 40 percent getting less exercise than they should.

4. **Keep your weight down and avoid obesity.** Today, nearly 40 percent of all Americans are considered obese, with obesity as a key factor in the increase of Type 2 Diabetes, which affects more than 12 million women. Even more dismaying is that children twelve to nineteen suffer a 20 percent obesity rate. Obesity is directly associated with high blood pressure, high cholesterol, and diabetes, all of which increase the risk for heart disease. Which is why it is so important to maintain a healthy body weight—one with a BMI <30 and a waist circumference of less than thirty-five inches—in order to prevent heart disease. Portion control is out of control, and so are our waistlines!

5. **Manage high lipid profile.** Keeping LDL (your bad cholesterol) low is the main way to control high cholesterol. Help keep that number down by increasing fresh fruits and vegetables, limiting saturated fats and salt—keep salt intake to less than 1 gram a day—reducing alcohol consumption, and increasing physical activity. Recommended levels of lipids include the following:

   * LDL <130mg/dl
   * HDL >50mg/dl
   * Triglycerides <150mg/dl (most common type of fat in the body)
   * Total cholesterol <200 mg/dl
   * Total cholesterol/HDL ratio should be below 5:1

6. **Blood pressure** should be less than 120/80mmHG. If your blood pressure readings are consistently greater than 130/80, medication may be recommended.
7. **Manage your stress.** It is well known that stress and stressors directly affect our health—just take a look at the Ornish diet recommendations. Stress not only affects our body physically, but it affects our emotions and behavior. Your reaction to stressful situations can be greatly influenced by healthy life choices, yoga, meditation, and the practice of mindfulness.
8. **Consider baby aspirin.** If you have any evidence of heart disease, a daily low dose aspirin (75mg daily) is recommended. Of course, as with taking any medication, over or behind the counter, check with your physician first.
9. **Include Omega 3-Fatty Acids.** These healthy fatty acids are best had by eating fatty fish and are recommended in order to help lower your risk of heart disease. The American Heart Association (AHA) recommends eating two 3.5-ounce servings of fatty fish—including salmon, albacore tuna, mackerel, herring, lake trout, and sardine—every week in order to reduce the risk of congestive heart failure, coronary heart disease, sudden cardiac arrest, and stroke. Unfortunately, Omega 3-fatty acid *supplements* have not proven to be as heart protective as originally thought. However, if you are healthy, but can't consume two servings of fish a week, for whatever reason, it's still recommended to take 250–500mg of Omega-3 (namely EPA and DHA-fish oil) every day. EPA and DHA are the *best* types of Omega-3 to take for optimal wellness, as studies point to their benefits in preventing cardiovascular

disease as well as cancer, asthma, depression, and rheumatoid arthritis.

10. **Alcohol...Friend or foe?** Drum roll, please. Here, especially, moderation is the key. For a healthy woman, *one drink a day* is recommended, while men may safely consume two drinks. Specifically, one drink means one serving of either a 5-ounce glass of wine, a 12-ounce beer or one 1.5-ounce shot of hard liquor**.** For you red wine drinkers: with all the hubbub about red wine's special antioxidants and flavonoids, the bad news is that it's not considered to be any more preventative against heart disease than red grape juice—which contains the same protective antioxidants without the negative effects of alcohol.
11. **Don't smoke.** Period. Don't use tobacco and try to avoid secondhand smoke. Cigarette smoking *triples* your risk of a heart attack.
12. **Get adequate amounts of sleep.** Every night. Ideally, a minimum of seven hours. You know how much you really need—whether it's six or ten. Sleep is so important.

Excitingly enough, we're living in a time when more and more women are being empowered to speak out and mobilize in order to fight injustice and inequity. We must use those same voices to encourage all women to educate themselves about their health risks and how to become proactive in reducing those risks.

The good news is that, since 1999, deaths from heart disease have fallen by about a third. A heart-healthy lifestyle gets the credit for this and demonstrates just how much influence one can have in reducing one's personal risk of heart disease.

## Hearty V

When it comes to heart disease, it is my hope that screening for the disease will become as important (and as standard) in a woman's yearly health care routine as mammograms and pelvic exams—beginning at age forty, at the very least.

As a proud ambassador for the American Heart Association and Go Red for Women—the Heart Association's national movement to end heart disease and stroke in women—it has been my mission to help educate women on the risks and prevention of this disease, and to empower them to take their heart health into their own hands. I look forward to the day when heart disease in women is nearly eliminated through action and awareness.

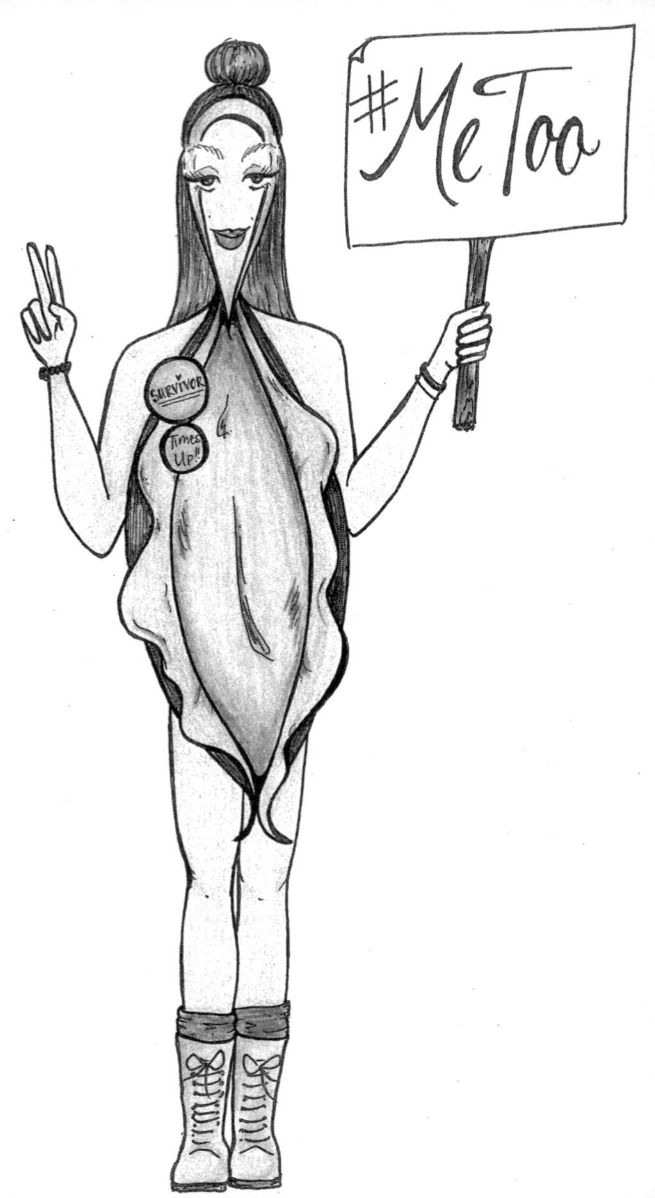
#MeToo
SURVIVOR
Times Up!!

CHAPTER 9

# #MeToo

"Although I grew up in a rural area of Georgia, I attended a public high school of nearly two thousand students. It was mostly an enjoyable experience, but there certainly wasn't much in the way of sex education. In fact, many of my peers dropped out due to teen pregnancy, so I think it's fair to say that a lot of kids were having sex.

However, I was still a virgin as I headed to college at Duke University, and the truth is, at the time, I was almost ashamed of that fact. Looking back, I realized that I simply wasn't ready until I was twenty. In hindsight, I also realized that every woman develops at a different pace.

After graduation from Duke, I moved to Los Angeles and started to make a career for myself as a model. I think I was taken by surprise by how quickly success came. With close to a million followers on Instagram, I found that young women were looking up to me, looking to me for tips about health and fitness.

I also became a patient of Dr. Sherry's. Frankly, I don't know what I would have done without her. It wasn't only that she taught more than I'd ever known about my own anatomy, she helped me through a situation that could have been potentially devastating. Unfortunately, it was a situation that countless other women have endured.

It happened that nude photos of me were leaked onto the internet. Someone had apparently hacked my ex-boyfriend's phone and released photos he'd *secretly* taken of me. And, of course, they weren't of me at dinner or at the beach, they were naked photos showing every part of my body. Most people I know do not want to show their vaginas to the world, but I did not have a choice. I had to find a way to deal with feelings that I'd been violated, which is where Dr. Sherry came in. She helped me realize that the female anatomy is not something to ever be ashamed of, and she kept me sane. Sure, it wasn't my decision to have those kind of pictures posted, but, because there will always be opportunistic and unscrupulous people, it's important to take charge and protect yourself.

If only sex education could undergo a complete overhaul across the country, and discussion about vaginas and sex weren't so awkward, if not completely taboo. To that end, Dr. Sherry is trying to crush those taboos and take the shame out of talking about what is probably one of the most important parts of a woman's anatomy. And thank goodness for that. ”

—**Elizabeth Turner** Model

I'm fairly certain Hannah Gadsby—of the phenomenal stand-up special *Nanette*—didn't set out to become a spokesperson for all things #MeToo and LGBTQ, rather, she very clearly did intend to set the record straight, in her unique and inimitable style, on homophobia and abuse, dysfunction, trauma, and toxic men. Her rendering of a life—her life—as an openly lesbian, activist, autistic, funny, angry comedian and former student of art history and curatorship (yes, she's all those things and more), in which she's encountered her unfair share of injustice, violence, discrimination, and homophobia strikes a nerve in everyone.

Until now, violence against women and the LGBTQ community, misogyny, shame, and self-deprecation have all been fertile sources of punch lines in comedy...and in life. Hannah manages to make us reflect on what a new, compassionate *normal* might be. In the wake of the #MeToo movement, she holds up a torch for all of us to see our way through the world.

## The Hypocrisy of the Hippocratic Oath to "Do No Harm"

As a women's health advocate and practicing OB-GYN for over twenty-five years, I feel it my duty to add to the conversation of sexual abuse by shining a light on a particular group of offenders that I find especially abhorrent—more so even than directors, actors, or clergymen—a group that not only has access to women in vulnerable situations, but also has the advantage of hiding behind a trusted and revered status. Sadly, I'm talking about doctors, including pediatricians, anesthesiologist, psychiatrists, and, especially, gynecologists. As small a percentage of medical professionals are included in this group, the dismaying fact is that these types of predators exist at all.

Fortunately, thanks to the #MeToo Movement, those doctors who have spent years abusing their position are finally knocking the usual suspects off the front pages of the newspapers. Case in point: Dr. Lawrence G. Nassar, the former team doctor for USA Gymnastics who was sentenced to 40 to 175 years in prison for sexually abusing more than 160 victims, some as young as six. Upon announcing Nassar's sentence, Judge Rosemarie Aquilina stated, "I just signed your death warrant." However, even though justice has been served to Dr. Nassar, the lives of his many victims will never be the same.

I have heard story upon story from my patients about sexual misconduct by doctors—misconduct that may have occurred *decades* earlier—that resulted in long-term effects both physically and emotionally. Many of these victims suffer posttraumatic stress disorders that have immobilized them throughout their lives.

Imagine this: You're sitting on an examination table in a small, brightly-lit room, completely naked except for a paper gown, nervously waiting for your new gynecologist to walk in and perform your first (or second or tenth) well woman exam. Maybe you selected this particular doctor from a list provided to you by your health insurer, or maybe he was recommended by an acquaintance. Either way, you may know relatively little about the man you're expecting to enter the examining room other than the fact that he'll probably be wearing a standard issue, white doctor's coat. That coat is emblematic in inspiring trust, just like a police officer's or fireman's uniform or, even—now, don't laugh—Superman's cape, Batman's mask, or Captain Marvel's sash and thunderbolt. The point is that you're seldom more *vulnerable,* or seldom expected to be as *trusting* as when you're half-naked in a doctor's office.

This is what one of my patients learned long before finding me:

*"There's no 'look' to a molester—doctor or otherwise. My molester was sixtyish, of average height and build, with close-cropped graying hair and an easy smile. He wore 'dad' slacks and Missoni sweaters and was my gynecologist. In one of his exam rooms he had a photo of a famous, thrice-divorced actress holding her infant son. On my first visit, I mentioned that I'd seen the actress in a recently released movie. His reply: 'Oh, I've done all her deliveries...as well as her abortions.' I know, I know, that should have been the tip-off for me. Instead, "dad slacks" became my regular gyno. The inappropriate behavior started slowly, with baby steps. Sometimes he would stay in the exam room 'doing paperwork' as I dressed to leave, and he would playfully smack my butt or tweak my boob. Red flags? Of course. I know that now, but, at the time, I was in an emotionally abusive relationship with a guy who had a similar 'sense of humor,' so I excused the behavior. As time went on, my molester ingratiated himself by sharing his personal and emotional history with me, in an attempt to make us feel more 'connected.' During one particular internal exam, with one hand inside me, he put his other hand down his corduroys...I went to the police shortly afterwards."*

Sexual misconduct accusations should be reported to each state's medical board to determine reprimands, but oftentimes violations are not reported, or, if they are, they're downplayed or swept under the umbrella of "unprofessional conduct," which is a catchphrase encompassing everything from sexual misconduct to the "crime" of inadequate record keeping. Beyond that, a doctor's license may only be revoked following a criminal conviction of their sexual misconduct. Even if an accusation does manage to result in a criminal conviction, only thirteen state medical boards actually notify their state or local law enforcements of a convicted doctor's sexual abuse. That's *thirteen out of fifty states*—a pathetic ratio, if you ask me.

Aside from feeling shame or embarrassment, many women don't report sexual misconduct because—believe it or not—they aren't certain of what, exactly, constitutes that misconduct. So just to be clear, "Sexual impropriety includes watching a patient undress, examining their genital areas without gloves, or *making inappropriate comments*. Sexual violations occur when a physician engages in physical sexual contact with the patient (such as kissing, sexual intercourse, or touching any sexualized body part for purposes outside an exam), offers drugs in exchange for sexual acts, masturbates in their presence, or encourages a patient to masturbate."

Know this for your own benefit, and for the benefit of a friend or family member who may confide in you about her own encounter with a doctor whose behavior didn't quite seem *kosher*. Also, in case you weren't already aware of exam protocol, it is customary for a male doctor to have a nurse or medical assistant present when he is performing an intimate exam. This protocol is also known as the "standard of practice," and, although it is required in only seven states for intimate exams by the American Medical Association (AMA)—which is the mother ship for doctors in the United States—it is certainly an important guideline for *most* doctors.

It doesn't seem possible, but, as of this writing, there are no nationally determined rules for "white coat" violators. The AMA does have a section in its constitution and bylaws called "Principles of Medical Ethics," which presents guidelines defining sexual harassment in the practice of medicine, but it stops short of outlining any disciplinary or legal actions.

That said, more and more medical professionals are working to help expose sexual predators in their particular fields and to hold them accountable for their actions. Esteemed physician, author, and medical historian, Dr. Howard Markel, recently noted, "The need for physicians to make a formal warrant of diligent, moral, and ethical conduct in the service of their patients may be stronger than ever." Might I also add how important it is for women to tell their stories of abuse, to not be afraid in this day and age of being judged or ridiculed or not being taken seriously. Women, tell your stories. Be silent no more, because the alternative may mean issues of lifelong stress and trauma, as I'd like to discuss further.

## Post-Traumatic Stress Disorder and Sexual Assault

> *"For thirty years, every time I imagined having my annual Pap smear, memories of my horrific first experience would start to surface."*

This is what Tanya told me one day as she shared with me her story of sexual assault at the hands of her first gynecologist; and, although the assault happened nearly thirty years prior during her very first intimate exam, even thinking about a Pap smear was enough to cause her to hyperventilate. Tanya continued:

> *"It was 1976 and I was sixteen. My parents were big donors to Cedars Sinai and UCLA Hospitals, so they were able to make an appointment for me with 'the best' OB-GYN. I felt pretty excited to be grown-up enough*

*to go for my first exam, and, of course, my mother felt assured that I was going to have the best possible care, so she waited in her car. I wasn't even nervous! Once my feet were in the stirrups and my front was draped with the paper sheath, the doctor came in with his nurse, but she only stayed for a moment because he told her, 'It's okay, you don't have to be here.' I didn't think anything of it because I didn't know any better. After she left, he started with the breast exam. He told me I had beautiful breasts and then his face came very close to mine. I remember the look of his rough skin and his long grey nose hairs as he came in closer. I didn't know what to expect, but then he said something like 'a little kiss doesn't hurt anything,' and he leaned down and kissed me hard on the mouth, sticking his tongue down my throat, his hands fondling my breasts. I don't remember anything else about the appointment except getting in my mother's car afterwards and telling her what happened. And this is the hard part; my mother said to me, 'Just don't tell anyone. Don't ever mention this to anyone. We'll get a new doctor.' And that was that. I never mentioned the story again. Until now, Dr. Sherry. Between the #MeToo movement and hearing Dr. Christine Ford bravely share her story, I felt it was my time, too, to release my dirty little secret. God, it feels good to share it."*

As many horror stories as the #MeToo Movement has uncovered, as many memories have resurfaced and as much trauma has been relived, it is far better than the silence and suppression that has gone on for years. For many women, that silence and suppression has been the cause of ongoing chronic stress and relationship problems in their lives. Emotional and physical intimacy has been sacrificed, as well as self-esteem and sanity. In order to end that cycle of trauma, women need to talk about their past abuse. It's a matter of health, well-being, and quality of life going forward.

While involved in a menopausal study examining hot flashes, Dr. Rebecca Thurston, a leading physician on cardiovascular risk and midlife women's health, found that 20 percent of the 304 women in the study had been sexually assaulted. Thurston went on to detail her findings, which suggested that sexual harassment and assault had a lasting and significant impact on the mental and physical health of midlife women. "Sexual harassment and assault are more than issues that impair a woman's quality of life and functioning. They also have implications for a woman's mental and physical health."

In presenting her findings at the North American Menopause Society's (NAMS) 2018 annual meeting, Thurston talked about the correlation of high blood pressure, sleep problems, and depression with sexual misconduct, and how prevention of such traumatic experiences as sexual abuse and misconduct has to be part of health promotion and disease prevention activities.

Post-Traumatic Stress Syndrome (PTSD) in women who have suffered sexual abuse is a real and ongoing crisis. The statistics are sobering:

A 2015 Centers for Disease Control and Prevention (CDC) data brief found:

* 43 percent of US women encounter some kind of sexual violence in their lives.
* More than 300,000 rapes are *reported* every year in the US.

* *Two thirds of rapes are never reported,* according to the Rape, Abuse & Incest National Network (RAINN). In fact, RAINN estimates that a sexual assault occurs in the US every ninety-eight seconds and "only six percent of the perpetrators of those attacks ever spend a day in jail—the lowest rate for any violent crime."

Each year, someone proclaims, "This is the year of the woman!" But what does that really mean? In fact, *The Year of the Woman* first appeared in headlines in 1992, after a *record number* of five women were elected to the US Senate. In response to that declaration, Senator Barbara Mikulski of Maryland—the longest-serving woman in the history of Congress—said, "Calling 1992 the Year of the Woman makes is sound like the Year of the Caribou or the Year of the Asparagus. We're not a fad, a fancy, or a year." *Touché.*

Take action; this year, this moment, at this time in your life. If you feel that a health care provider has inappropriately touched you, I implore you to do the following:

* Do NOT remain silent.
* Talk to someone who is trustworthy about the incident.
* Contact the National Sexual Assault Telephone Hotline 800-656-HOPE (4673).
* Report the incident to the state medical board and create a police report.
* Contract SNAP (Survivors Network of those Abused by Priests), a support and advocacy organization for people sexually abused by doctors, therapists, clergy, and others.
* Find a therapist you can confide in who has the credentials and experience to help you deal with trauma.

As Hannah Gadsby so eloquently put it: "There is nothing stronger than a broken woman who has rebuilt herself."

With that said, I feel it's my duty to do what I can to help prevent abuse from happening in the first place. After all, there's not much good in stating the problem if you can't try to offer a solution. That's like giving an eloquent lecture on the dangers of contracting, say, tuberculosis and what symptoms to look for, without including ways to *avoid* contracting the disease in the first place. Such as it is with disease, it's so helpful to be *informed* in regard to how to prevent and avoid acts of sexual misconduct. You may start by understanding the difference between what is appropriate—when in the vulnerable position of being in a doctor's exam room—and what is *not* appropriate. For that, I give you:

## How to Inform Your V

Right about now, I hope you're asking, "What can I do to prevent sexual misconduct during a visit with a health care provider?" So what I'd like to examine first is the way in which to choose a provider—specifically, an OB-GYN—in the first place. It's amazing how many women assume that, just because someone has gone to medical school, that person is immune to abusive or hypocritical behavior. Just as you would ask around—or take it to the "hive mind" on Facebook or Instagram—in order to find a good mechanic or caterer or fitness instructor, you must do the same when looking for an OB-GYN.

I understand that most of us are given a list of providers to choose from in accordance with our medical insurance companies, but that is no excuse to forego your research. Between social media, Yelp, reputable physician review sites, and word of mouth, you may learn about doctors and what their patients past and present have thought of them. Interview your potential OB-GYN once you've landed on one—or two or three. The most important aspect is that you feel *comfortable* talking openly and honestly with the person in front of you. If you find that you don't feel comfortable or you just don't like the vibe of a particular doctor, don't feel obliged to go to him (or her) just because you've taken their time or because you've "already made an appointment and *feel bad* canceling." Listen, you don't feel embarrassed or obliged to buy a dress that doesn't fit—or maybe you do, and that's not good either—so why should you feel that way when the fit doesn't feel right between you and a potential doctor? Find someone with whom you feel at ease. That is the first step.

If you decide on a new *male* OB-GYN, at the time of your exam, you shouldn't hesitate to request that a female chaperone (usually, the doctor's nurse) be present in the exam room for your visit. In fact, you ought never to be alone in an exam room with a male OB-GYN. Having taken these early precautions, you might think, "I'm done. Whatever happens now is just going to be routine." But sometimes we're not in a position—literally or figuratively—to know what constitutes *routine*. Case in point is my patient, Katie, who shared with me a story from her first pregnancy. Unfortunately, it is not an unusual story and should fall under the category of what *not* to expect when you're expecting:

> *"When I was in early labor in my first pregnancy, the doctor on call from my OB-GYN group was summoned to do a cervical check on me for dilation. The entire time, he was performing the check, he also happened to*

*be applying steady pressure to my clitoris. At the time, I thought maybe it was accidental or maybe it was the only way to position his hand or maybe he was trying to distract my attention from the pain of a cervical check. When I asked people in my birth group if anyone had had the same experience, the answer was a unanimous 'No!' They said that any doctor doing a cervical check would know where a clitoris is and whether or not they were on it. Besides, one of the first things an OB-GYN is taught is to be careful of touching a woman's clitoris—and any accidental touch should warrant an apology. Even if the touch was being used as a distraction, it could be categorized as assault. All I remember was that the touch was purposeful—even though my husband and a nurse were in the room—and the doctor was unapologetic. My response during the exam was to act as if I didn't notice, especially since everyone else in the room seemed blithely unaware of what was happening. I was embarrassed to say anything, and I was worried that I'd embarrass the doctor, so I stayed quiet about it. Four years later, I had a different doctor for my second birth. Needless to say, that doctor never came anywhere close to touching my clitoris, which is when I realized that it's not normal routine to do so. Four years after the fact, I filed a complaint to the medical group, but found myself giving the doctor the benefit of the doubt—again. I had a hard time believing his intent was sexually motivated because I couldn't imagine how a medical professional could do such a thing. Even though I've since been told that what he did was inappropriate, I can't help but think that maybe it really was a medical necessity or an accident. I don't know if he's done anything like that to anyone else. I mean, I still hear good things about him.*

*He's well liked. Hell, I liked him as a doctor until that incident because he seemed kind and was generous with his time in addressing my questions and concerns; more so than the other doctors in his group."*

I can't repeat this often enough: First off, you must have a nurse or chaperone in the exam room with you during an exam with a male OB-GYN. And, even then, if you have any uncomfortable feelings during the exam, or you feel unsafe at any time, speak out immediately to the nurse and then to the office manager. Afterward, any inappropriate activity should be reported to the medical board in your particular state.

There are plenty of things *not* to expect when visiting an OB-GYN, which is why it may be helpful now to let you know exactly what you may expect.

## What to Expect During Your OB-GYN Exam

Especially with a brand new OB-GYN, there may be some nerves on that first visit. Those nerves may be compounded if this is your first well woman or OB-GYN visit ever! It's a good idea to have your paperwork emailed ahead of time so that you can get it out of the way in order to avoid being overwhelmed by it at the time of your visit. So now you can just show up and not feel as if you've just been assigned an unwelcome homework assignment—yes, I know the paperwork can be a drag, but it is ultimately helpful. Then, even if you assume the doctor is running late, arrive a little early just so you have time to decompress from the day, the traffic, and your deadlines. Relax. Bring a book or sit back and listen to some of your favorite tunes. I'm serious. We forget that waiting rooms are a perfect excuse to take advantage of a little free time. Even

I have to wait when I see my own doctor or dentist or chiropractor! If you need some extra comfort, maybe you can find that comfort in numbers. Bring your BFF, your sister, or your mother along. They can hold your hand literally and figuratively in the waiting room and during your well woman exam.

Ah, yes, *the well woman exam.* You've heard it mentioned, but what exactly is it, and what does it entail?

The standard well woman exam refers to the most common visit you'll make to your OB-GYN. If this is your first visit with this particular doctor, you may first go into the doctor's office in order to have a discussion about your medical history or any concerns you may have, although some doctors have this conversation in the exam room prior to the examination. After your conversation in the office, the doctor's nurse will usually greet you and take your blood pressure and ask you to hop on the scale. Though not every well woman exam involves a urine sample, it is pretty standard procedure to be asked for one. After all that, you will find yourself in the actual exam room.

Upon entering the room, you'll be asked to remove all your clothing, including bra and underwear, don one of those lovely, disposable paper gowns—one size fits all—and have a seat on the examination table. Most gowns consist of a top that opens in the front along with a separate paper blanket that drapes over your waist and vagina. After you've changed, the first person to enter is usually the nurse or medical assistant—sometimes blood pressure is taken at this time, instead of earlier. Finally, your doctor enters. He may first check your thyroid gland, which is located in the front middle part of your neck, and then he'll listen with a stethoscope to your heart and lungs.

All along, you doctor ought to be explaining what he is doing or about to do, such as: “I’m checking your thyroid.” Or, “I’m going to listen to your heart and lungs now.” After those preliminary checks, standard procedure is to do a breast exam.

For the breast exam, you’ll be asked to lay flat back on the table. If your doctor is starting with your right breast, you’ll be asked to put your right arm over your head—conversely, left breast, left arm overhead. Your doctor will use the pads of his fingers to check for lumps or tenderness by gently pressing down and moving his fingers in a manner that covers every quadrant of breast tissue and underarm lymph nodes. Afterward, he will usually check your nipples by gently squeezing to make sure that there is no discharge coming from the area.

Once your breast exam is done, your doctor will check your abdominal area. Using his hands, he may press or palpitate the area under the liver, which is located in the upper right side of your abdomen. The lower abdominal area is pressed or palpitated in much the same way in order to feel for any masses or tenderness.

Last—and certainly not least—the pelvic exam, where you’ll be asked to put your feet in the silver stirrups at the end of the table. We doctors tend to use the same, decidedly nonmedical term “scooch,” as in, “Please scooch down,” which means that you are to bring your butt to the edge of the table so that your knees are bent toward the ceiling. With your paper blanket draped over your waist and pelvic area, the doctor will take a seat between your legs. He’ll then push back the paper to uncover your vulva and vagina.

Your doctor may then check for any abnormalities that may be obviously visible. With sterile gloves on—usually latex, unless you know you have a particular allergy to latex—

he may touch the vulvar area if there is anything that seems visually concerning. A speculum is then inserted into your vagina in order to inspect the inside and have eyes on your cervix. It should be noted here that speculums come in a few sizes in order to accommodate those who become squeamish or experience pain with a regular-sized speculum. You can ask your doctor to use a smaller speculum during your pelvic exam if, for any reason, you're uncomfortable with the one she is using. Once your cervix is identified, the speculum is tightened in place in order to perform a Pap smear. In order to do a Pap smear, delicate instruments called brushes and brooms are used to gently scrape and collect cervical and endocervical cell samples. During the Pap smear, the broom is used to sweep the face of the cervix and then the brush is used to collect the sample. Both the broom and brush are then placed in a sterile container so that they can be sent to a pathology lab in order to be tested. That finished, the speculum is removed, and a bimanual exam is performed.

In the bimanual exam, the doctor will insert his gloved index and middle finger inside your vagina while his opposite hand is placed on your lower abdominal area. The two fingers are used to palpate the cervix in order for the opposite hand to check for masses or abnormalities in the uterus and ovaries. Depending on your age, you may also be down for one more bit of probing, the rectal exam, which is performed by the insertion of *one*—thank goodness—gloved finger in your anus. If you're over fifty, you can pretty much count on this last check. And, of course, you should follow up with that baseline colonoscopy if you're fifty or older!

Time to take a breath, because you're basically done. At this point, it's time for your doctor to snap off the gloves and say something to the effect of "See you next year!" Most times, that's what happens. You ought to get your test results from your labs and Pap smear in the mail in the coming weeks, and, unless something seems amiss, you'll have a year until you have to do the whole thing over.

But what if you've decided, for one reason or another—perhaps you're not crazy about your doctor's "bedside manner," or she/he is retiring, or you've been feeling rushed or ignored at regular visits, or you're changing insurance plans and your current doctor is not on your new plan—you need to find a new doctor? Or what if you need to find your *first* OB-GYN *ever*?

For you, I have:

## The Best Approach to Finding a New Doctor

These days, most women are given a list of doctors to choose from by their insurance provider, so that's usually a starting point. Between social media, Yelp, physician review sites—of which there are at least a half dozen—you should be able to whittle down your choices. But don't stop there. Once you find a couple potential doctors, you can always interview them before committing to an office visit. Depending on what's most important to you in an OB-GYN, you may want to choose some (or all) of the following questions to ask:

1. Will I get a call back with my test results? Do you email or mail the results?
2. Will you be calling me back or will it be one of your office staff members?
3. Are you accessible via email?
4. How far in advance must I book an appointment? What about if it's an emergency?

5. How often do you suggest I have a Pap smear?
6. What are your views on mammograms?

The most important question is the one you have to answer yourself: Do I feel comfortable talking openly and honestly with this person?

If you think you've landed on "the one," it's a good idea to make sure your potential OB-GYN is board-certified and there are no malpractice claims against him or her.

For girls under the age of twenty-one—and it's recommended that girls start to see an OB-GYN between the ages of *thirteen and fifteen* in order for them to start building a long-term relationship and to discuss sexually transmitted infections, prevention, and other health care issues—the good news is that your first visit may only consist of a *conversation*. Unless you're sexually active or have vaginal discharge or pain, or any other complaints about what's happening "down south," you will not need an internal pelvic exam, not yet.

Pap smears, which obviously do involve an internal exam, are not routine until the age of twenty-one.

Don't wait to find an OB-GYN until something is wrong, when you might be forced to pick a name—any name—out of a proverbial hat. Your relationship with your OB-GYN should be based on the long term. I'm now delivering the babies of girls that I delivered! Start with a relationship that feels comfortable. Choose a doctor that you've researched and interviewed and have no qualms about asking important or seemingly embarrassing questions. And, if you ever feel that your doctor has crossed a line, never ever try to convince yourself that it's okay, or that it's all in your head, or that it's probably a one-time deal. From what you've read here, I hope you now know otherwise.

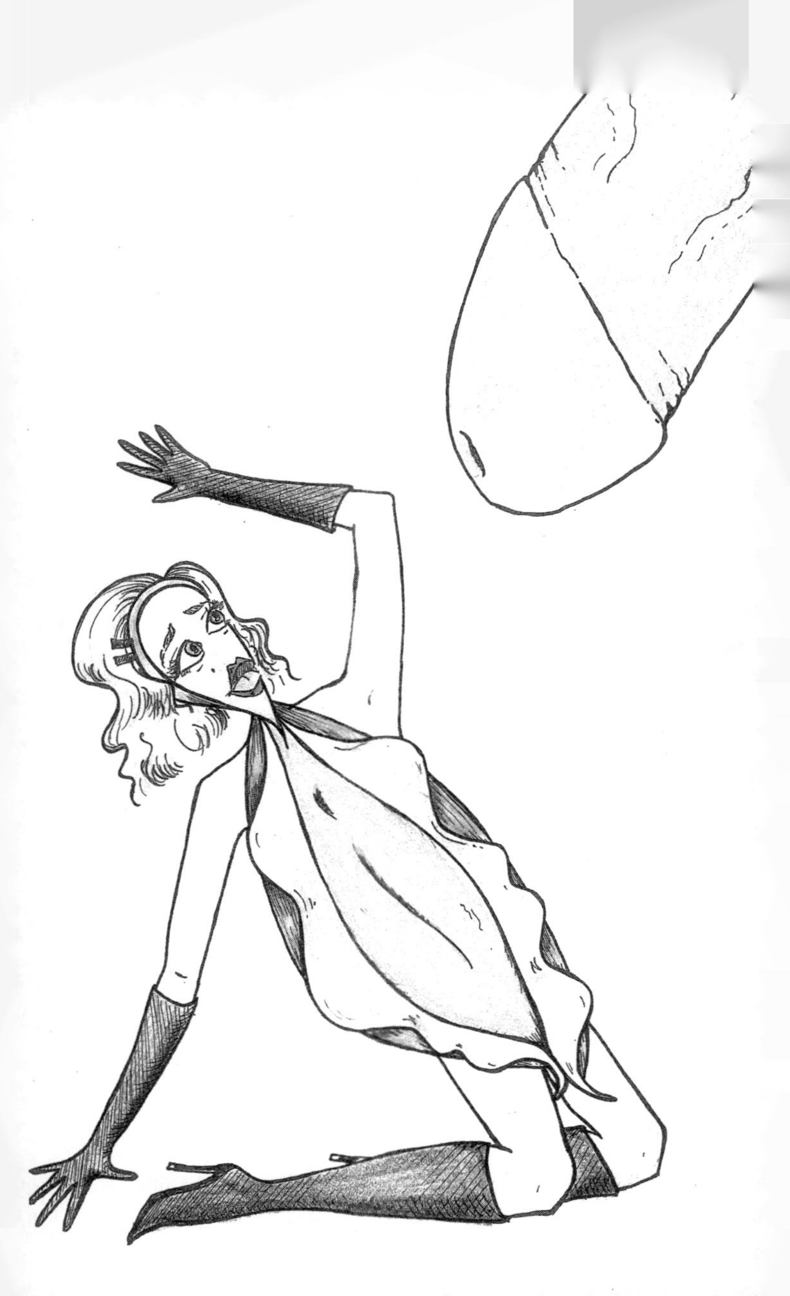

## CHAPTER 10

# TLC

"I am a gay woman, (Surprise, Mom. I *did* have my name engraved on my tackle box. You do the gay math.) so penis size was never something I thought much about unless I was shopping for a dilda. (I've always called it a 'dilda' because it just sounds so much classier than 'dildo.' And it's the feminine version of the noun that comes from 'dildar,' meaning 'to park it up in there.'

There *was* a two-year hetero stint I had in my mid-twenties after my first girlfriend. I called it 'My Stroll Down Penis Avenue.' It wasn't a bang-a-thon, but I slept with a few good men. One man had the largest penis I had ever seen, and I ride horses. It was fascinating like fireworks in that you wanted to stare at it for the whole show, but didn't want it too close to your face. I spent an evening with that penis and its jockey and it was not only painful, but it wouldn't stay in. I remember thinking, 'Wow, so much talk about large weens being the brass ring, but that thing was just unusable.' When I woke up in the morning I remember feeling like I had experienced a highly inaccurate bounce on a pogo stick. It was what I called a very bad 'wangover,' even though I think that's a pot term. I don't know. I'm still on AOL, guys. Be gentle.

A couple years later, on my thirtieth birthday, my friend bought me a dilda that was just enormous. Like when people get you those giant "joke" cookies with your name frosted on it that are the size of a record album. You know you're not gonna eat it, but you like having it around. It was very pricey, and, as dildas go, a work of art. So realistic and included two bonus balls and a suction cup. I remember sticking it to the wall when friends would come over for the laugh. One morning, my friend put it on my mantle right before the bug man came to spray my house. It was a great comedy prop.

The reason I'm talking about said huge dilda is because I don't know how or when or how long it took, but I very gradually worked up to using it. I was pretty sensitive and prone to pain if something was big, but I found out that the young and mighty malleable vagina is a thing of wonder. With enough patience, the right music, and hips that can unhinge like a snake's jaw, anything is possible. I mean, baby heads come out of there by the millions. It made me understand how a boa constrictor can look at a massive deer and be like, 'Maybe... worth a shot.'

As I have gotten older (I'm forty-thirteen), I have dealt with a sharp increase in pain from penetration. It's not pleasant and it was great to feel comfortable enough with Dr. Sherry to discuss it at length. She pulled that mirror out and started explaining all the possible issues that might be causing me pain. It was one of the best dates I've ever been on, although I think everyone at PF Chang's was traumatized. I did realize how much we as women just file things under the generic 'something hurts down there' and rarely get to the root of the problem.

As Eleanor Roosevelt once said to a tree after nine drinks, 'Life is far too short to have pain in the dilda garage.' ”

—**Paula Pell** Comedy Writer, Producer, and Actress

## Bigger but Not Necessarily Better

You heard that right. And, yes, we're going to get right into it, but I will let Monica, an acerbically funny patient of mine with a new boyfriend—and a new dilemma—give this introduction:

Monica, at her last exam: *"He has the biggest dick I have ever seen! It's not just longer than a regular penis, it's as thick as my freakin' fist. It's like I'm having sex with a Snapple bottle! Every time we have sex, I'm in pain and I wind up with tears on the outside of my LaLa. What do I do?"*

*Oh, Monica!* To be fair, the penis has its own share of nicknames to rival those of the vagina: One-Eyed Monster, Spitting Cobra, Yingyang, Dong...the list goes on. And, certainly, some of those names are not for nothing—case in point: Deep V Diver.

If, after a few drinks, a dinner party conversation happens to veer into the territory of penis size, it usually has to do with jokes about *small,* unfulfilling-sized members. Truthfully, I never hear people talk about the terrible nature of an anaconda-sized penis—even among girlfriends on a Friday night Happy Hour. But, when it comes to causing actual pain, a bigger than average penis is no laughing matter.

Just like the vagina and labia, the penis and scrotum come in all sizes (and shapes). The smallest penis on record is 1 centimeter (.39 inches), the longest, 34 centimeters (13.5

inches)—*no comment*. The *typical* penis is an average of 5.7 inches long and 4.8 inches in diameter (girth). A vagina will stretch and acclimate to the size of a particularly large penis, but it may take time and patience.

Popular media would have us believe that bigger is, indeed, better, and that the very definition of masculinity lies in penis size. Advertisers want to convince men and women alike that this is so. In truth, penis size is not very high on a women's list of priorities when it comes to sexual partners. Rather, honesty, sense of humor, and affection are traits that rank higher than penis size. However, given a choice of length versus girth, women do generally prefer a thicker rather than a longer penis, the argument being that girth is helpful in experiencing the sense of "fullness" which leads to a successful orgasm. But that feeling of "fullness" can be strained to the point of discomfort and pain when a partner has an unusually large penis. In fact, vaginal tearing from an overly large penis is one of the most painful and challenging conditions to treat. While the vagina is very forgiving after a vaginal delivery, tears due to a plus-size penis require a long road to recovery.

First things first: If you are experiencing discomfort based on the size of your partner's penis, it's important to make your feelings known at the beginning of your relationship. If you're having problems, chances are that a previous partner or two of his has had the same problem. A good time to broach the subject of a pain-inducing-sized member would definitely be outside of the sexual experience and in a manner that is gentle and supportive.

Some things to remember if you do wind up with a partner like Monica's:

* Open, honest communication between you and your partner is key.
* Adequate lubrication is equally important—even if you think you naturally have enough, you can't go wrong with some extra KY.
* Avoid positions of deep penetration.
* Take it slow!
* Try topical lidocaine at the entrance of the vagina prior to intercourse.
* Consider using vaginal dilators or a dildo to increase the entrance size of the vagina.

And, by the way, there is no perfect penis. In fact, it was found that attention to cosmetic appearance—referring to cleanliness, trimmed pubic hair, and even "man-scaping"—was the most important consideration in a desirable penis!

## Other Causes of Vaginal Pain

As mentioned in detail in the **Cranky V** chapter from my first book, *She-ology: The Definitive Guide to Women's Intimate Health. Period.*, there are many common vulvar irritants, such as soaps, creams, and rubber products (to name just a few) that can cause pain and/or itchiness in and around the vagina. Some of those irritants may also lead to chronic medical conditions that require treatment. The good news is that many of those irritants can be easily avoided once recognized as culprits.

Aside from those conditions in **Cranky V**, there are the STIs of **Benched V**—also discussed in length in my first book—which are not only painful but may also be life-threatening if left undiagnosed and untreated. Here in the remainder of this chapter, we'll look take a look at other possible causes of a TLC V.

You may not know it, but clitoral and vulvar pain are very common in women, yet it's often difficult for doctors to treat such pain, including clitorodynia (which refers to pain of the clitoris) simply because women don't know enough themselves about the clitoris. Seriously, one third of university-aged women can't even locate the clitoris on an anatomically correct diagram. As I spoke about earlier, most women use code or slang when referring to their own "lady parts." Even certain slang terms for female reproduction organs connote derogatory terms—*pussy* refers to a weakling, *cunt* to an unpleasant person (rather, people ought to genuflect to these terms!). Given the evidence suggesting that one's sense of *body ownership* may influence one's sense of pain, it's no surprise that a *lack of clitoris ownership* (or, perhaps, a lack of clitoris pride) may be the reason for the prevalence of conditions such as clitorodynia.

### Lichen Sclerosis (LS)

One of the most disruptive and chronic conditions involving the vulva is called Lichen (pronounced *like-in*) Sclerosis, which represents nearly 40 percent of skin disorders.

With LS, the skin of the vulva becomes ivory or white, like the color of cigarette paper or parchment, and is accompanied by intense itching, burning, and pain. Intercourse and urination may also be a source of discomfort and pain, although a small percentage of patients do not have any symptoms at all. Most commonly seen in women forty to fifty years of age, LS can affect any age group. No one is certain as to what causes Lichen Sclerosis, but we do know that it is not contagious.

Diagnosis is made by examination and a biopsy of a small patch of the affected area.

Unfortunately, Lichen Sclerosis is incurable, but the symptoms are treatable. Therefore, treatment of this chronic condition is first and foremost about educating oneself on how to properly *manage* those symptoms.

Powerful steroid creams are usually used to control the symptoms but can only be used for a limited period of time, since they can further thin the delicate skin of the vulva. Initial treatment includes the use of steroid cream once or twice daily for three months. Thereafter, tapering the steroid cream will help reduce further complications. Meanwhile, there are methods of hydrating and caring for your skin while the creams take effect, methods that should be part of your daily feminine hygiene routine. They include:

- Removing potential skin irritants from use, such as detergents and fragrant soaps.
- Taking frequent baths with extra virgin coconut oil or Aveeno baths to hydrate the skin.
- Using olive oil, extra virgin coconut oil, or shortening as moisturizers.
- Using skin protectants such as A & D ointment or KY jelly, especially with sexual intercourse.
- Avoiding tight-fitting clothing such as pantyhose and jeans (silk underwear is recommended over cotton).

Untreated LS can lead to other serious problems including vulvodynia (see below), and may increase your risk of squamous cell carcinoma of the affected area. If appropriate and persistent daily care and treatment of the vulva is followed, this disruptive skin disorder won't get the better of you.

## *Vulvodynia*

Vulvodynia is an extremely painful condition involving the vulva and vagina, the causes of which are unidentifiable. Symptoms include burning, stinging, itching, throbbing, swelling, and soreness—an agonizing, disruptive recipe, to be sure. For an added one-two punch, these symptoms are chronic, come without warning and last a variable amount of time. Exercise, tampon insertion, the ability to wear jeans, sexual intercourse, and various other everyday activities can become impossible with the onset of this condition.

What we do know is that there are some influences associated with vulvodynia, such as infection, hormonal changes related to the menstrual cycle, spasms of the vagina muscles, vaginal nerve damage, history of sexual abuse, and chemical allergies. Diagnosis can be very difficult, since the vulvar area may appear completely normal upon examination. Usually, diagnosis is done via a thorough medical history along with a cotton-swab test, during which pressure is applied to various vulvar sites.

Treatment varies from person to person and may include a combination of methods, which may last from weeks to months. During this time, general self-care of the vulva is vital, as is true when dealing with any problems down south. In fact, most of these tips are interchangeable with the ones in **Cranky V**, but they bear repeating.

### *Self-Care Tips*

- Keep the vulva clean by using warm water and gentle patting. Rinse and pat dry the vulva after urination.
- Avoid rubbing the vulva, especially when bathing.

* Avoid perfumed soap or scented toilet paper.
* Avoid douching, feminine sprays, or talcum powder.
* Avoid pads or tampons that contain deodorant or plastic coating.
* Avoid pantyhose, unless it has a cotton crotch.
* Avoid tight-fitting pants or underwear.
* Use adequate lubrication during intercourse.

Non-medical treatment includes icepacks, cool gel packs, and Vaseline to relieve the pain and swelling. Pelvic floor physical therapy, vaginal dilators, biofeedback, dietary changes, and couple and sexual counseling have also been utilized in treating vulvodynia.

Topical medical treatments may include lidocaine 2.5 percent ointment (a local anesthetic), for use especially before sexual contact (applied thirty minutes prior). Other numbing ointments that have been proven successful are Emla cream, LMX 4 percent cream, and topical estrogen.

Oral medications include antidepressants such as Amitriptyline, Nortriptyline, and Prozac and anticonvulsants such as gabapentin and carbamazepine (which are also used to treat neuropathic pain). In the case of unbearable and unrelenting symptoms, surgery is often a last resort.

Truly, vulvodynia is a confusing and frustrating medical condition for both the health care provider and patient. Emotional and psychological support goes hand-in-hand with medical treatment options.

*Jane started as my patient when she was twenty-eight. A virginal, sweetly innocent, and strict Catholic, she planned on maintaining her virginity until marriage. I happened to be her first gynecologist, which, naturally, meant that I performed her first pelvic exam—an external one. Jane could not abide even a mini-speculum near her vagina and had never used a tampon. I respected, perhaps a bit grudgingly, her choice not to have an internal exam. Though, when Jane expressed her hopes to have children someday, I had to bite my tongue—what I wanted to say was "Children? How about sex?" When she came in for a vaginal itch or discharge, which wasn't very often, she wouldn't let me put a Q-tip into her vagina. When it did come time for her yearly pelvic exam, she would tense up, close her knees and nearly propel herself off the table. This went on for six years. Finally, to her credit, Jane went to the counseling I'd recommended to try and understand her reluctance. Originally, I had asked her if she'd ever been raped or molested. No and no, she'd replied. Another two years went by. Jane appeared for a yearly visit bursting with the news that she had met a wonderful man named David on Catholicsoulmates.com. Seven months later, they were married. Jane came in to my office shortly afterwards. "We want to get pregnant soon," she told me, "but the only problem is that I can only have anal sex. Vaginal sex is impossibly painful." So I met with Jane and David together and we discussed strategies to ease Jane into vaginal sex. Within six months, they were able to have sex with vaginal finger penetration. In six more, they were able to finally direct David's sperm in the right direction! After two years of marriage and an abundance of patience, understanding, and a willingness to make change, Jane was pregnant with her first child!*

## *Vaginismus*

A showstopper if ever there was one, vaginismus is an unusual condition which causes the muscles of the vaginal opening to tighten, making sexual intercourse and pelvic examination painful to the point of impossible. The treatment for vaginismus may include a combination of psychotherapy, relaxation exercises, physical therapy, vaginal dilators, and vaginal exercises allowing a finger or safe, sterile object to be inserted into the vagina. Ironically, the goal is a de-sensitization of sorts in order to allay the patient's fear of vaginal entry.

With patience, acceptance, and aggressive therapy, vaginismus can be successfully treated.

## *Hidradenitis Suppurativa (HS)*

Hidradenitis Suppurativa—not so affectionately known as HS—is a condition wherein the hair follicles of the vulva and vaginal area become blocked, swollen, inflamed and tender, resulting in painful lumps under the skin. Those lumps can then burst, forming painful "tunnels" under the skin. HS can be found any place on the body where there are hair follicles, including the armpits, groin, buttocks, and breasts.

Although the cause of HS is not fully understood, genetic and environmental factors are known to play a part in this painful condition. What we do know about HS is this:

* Women are more likely to get HS than men.
* One is more likely to contract HS if a family member has had it.
* Obesity and tobacco use may make you more susceptible to HS.

* Symptoms of HS are more commonly discovered after the age of puberty, but before the age of 30.
* HS is not contagious.
* HS has nothing to do with poor hygiene.
* Medication and surgery is often the best way to treat HS.

Most important in treating this chronic, embarrassing, and painful skin condition of the vulva and vagina, is finding a dermatologist who has experience managing HS and its symptoms.

## *Painful Orgasms, the Ultimate Bitter Sweet*

Pain with orgasm is probably more common than most woman really want to admit. Causes of painful orgasms include lack of adequate lubrication, vulvar or clitoral irritants such as soaps, creams, and rubber products, rough sex, vulvar skin conditions such as Lichen Sclerosis, and vaginal dryness due to menopause.

In addition to painful orgasms, you may also experience excruciating pain during sex, which I cover in depth in the **Collapsed V**. Such pain may be caused by vaginal dryness, vaginal infections, vaginal tears, latex allergy, ruptured ovarian cyst, endometriosis, vaginismus, emotional problems such as anxiety, and a history of sexual abuse, or may be due to a particular positioning during sex.

In order to address and treat these conditions, it's important not only to meet with a health care professional, it's imperative that you be honest and open about your sexual experiences with that health care professional. You have to make your sexual health a priority, and, to do that, you must be able to describe, in detail, what's going on with your body and when and where you feel any pain.

Painful conditions of the vulva and vagina are not discussed nearly as often as necessary. Many of my colleagues either haven't the time to review the care necessary for a painful vagina or their patients don't think it an important enough problem to bring up. Health care professionals need to directly address this problem in order for women to navigate treatment plans. If yours doesn't, or you don't feel comfortable with a prescribed treatment, please don't hesitate to get a second or third opinion. Find out what's making that vagina of yours so sensitive to pain.

*Do not* let pain ruin your intimacy or your life. As with Jane, the thing to overcome was fear itself!

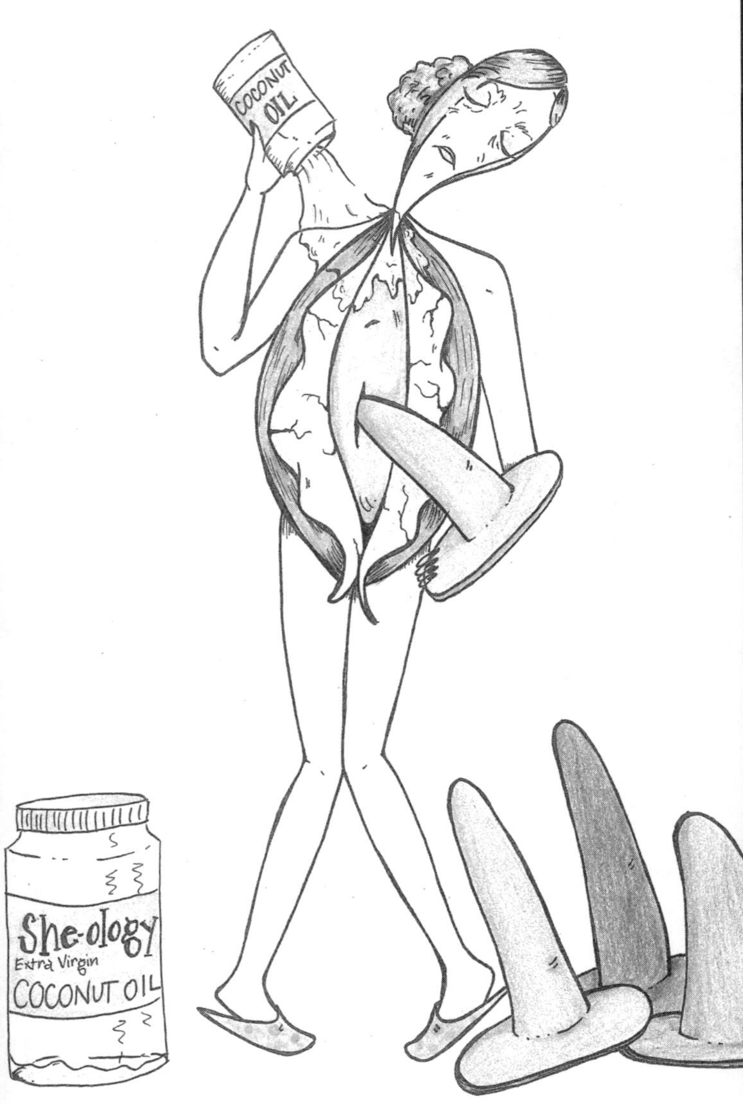
COCONUT OIL
She-ology
Extra Virgin
COCONUT OIL

## CHAPTER 11

# collapsed

"Most of my sexual health knowledge came from those awkward Sex Ed classes we all had to endure when we were too young to take seriously the exercise of putting a condom on a banana, let alone grasp the importance of such an education. While words like *vas deferens* and *seminal vesicles* still don't mean much to me (although I vaguely remember them having to do with testicles) I'm sure there was a lot of information that would have come in handy, had I been mature enough to absorb it or had I been given it in a more intimate setting by someone I felt comfortable with.

Unfortunately, I associate my early sexual health education with shame and embarrassment, and there's nothing healthy about that! It didn't help that my very modest mother felt equally embarrassed talking about sex.

Ironically, because my mother had a cancer scare when I was thirteen, she managed to further my sexual education in one essential way. She made sure I received the Gardasil immunization shots for HPV. I'd never heard of HPV, let alone known of anyone immunized, so I didn't understand the urgency. Fortunately, because I was young, I did what Mom said.

(Now, over fifteen years later, I'm glad I did, because I know how common and dangerous HPV is for women. Sadly, I know of more women my age with HPV than women that were immunized. Coincidence? I think not. So, even though my mom avoided talk about everything else sex-related, she did give me that!)

Despite a lack of sex education in school, I knew that STDs or pregnancy could easily halt my big plans for future success and independence. So, when I decided to lose my virginity to my high school boyfriend, he and I planned out the *entire event* well in advance. We knew the date, the place, and the methods of birth control and protection we would use! We knew the class to skip in order to visit a walk-in clinic for my prescription for the pill—and how far in advance I needed to start taking it in order to ensure its highest effectiveness. We were possibly the two most responsible virgins ever to plan their de-flowering.

Since moving to L.A. on my own, right after high school, Dr. Ross has been my gynecologist as well as one of the few permanent fixtures in my adult life. When I became pregnant a decade after that move, Dr. Ross treated my husband and me as much more than patients. Without any family in town, she patiently answered all our first-time (paranoiac) pregnancy questions and made us feel safe. She did that and much more, making every appointment exciting and laughter-filled.

When it came time for delivery, I endured eighteen hours of labor before being told I needed a C-section. That was one of my biggest fears, so much so that I never even factored that possibility into my birth plans. I was so panicked I could barely catch my breath between frightened sobs. Dr. Ross cleared my hospital room and looked me straight in eye. She calmly told me it was all right to cry, but that my baby needed a C-section, and I was strong enough to handle it. My hysteria abated, and I immediately summoned a 'Let's do this!' attitude. Moments later, I was wheeled into the OR.

Thanks, in large part, to Dr. Ross, I met my baby girl as the strong, resilient mama I'd wanted to be for her from the beginning. My gratitude for Dr. Ross is boundless. Aside from being the best damn doctor ever, she's one of the best damn humans as well. Truly. ”

—**Shenae Grimes-Beech** Actress

When I think about how easy it has been for society to marginalize the **aging vagina**, I can almost believe that God really is a man! However, with so many women-centric advancements taking root, many of which have sprung up from the #MeToo movement, I'm finding that women's sexual health is finally taking a front—if not exactly center—seat in the spotlight. If I may, I'd like to take that spotlight and shine it a little closer to the issue of sexual health for women over fifty. "Older vaginas" are still in need of a voice—so to speak—and I'm here to give it to them, as are a number of other qualified and enthusiastic physicians and educators, one of which is Dr. Sheryl Kingsberg.

As president of the North American Menopause Society (NAMS)—yes, there really is a national menopause society—Dr. Kingsberg has said, "With the recognition that women have a right to their sexual health, it's important to make our membership (referring to other OB-GYNs) comfortable with the dialogue about it." She and many other health professionals are aware of what a difficult time older women have in talking about their sexual health, especially as it relates to the vagina. Although vaginal dryness, painful sex, and inability to orgasm are some of the key issues for women over fifty, those are the very issues that women and their doctors seem most uncomfortable talking about. Look, doctors are people—and they are certainly not mind readers—which often means that they are as uncomfortable as their female patients in having the *mature* sex talk. The sad fact remains that 40 percent of women do not share sexually related problems with their health care providers. And since those providers do not open up the conversations in the first place, so much pertinent information about sexual dysfunction goes unsaid.

In her attempts to re-educate OB-GYNs and other health care providers, Dr. Kingsberg has nailed the definition of sexual dysfunction as a "loss of wanting to want." This simple re-defining of the term "sexual dysfunction" helps guide treatment in the direction of "focusing on the desire for desire as much as achieving sexual satisfaction," which is key for treating women—especially since women's sexual desire, unlike men's, tends to begin in that great organ *above the shoulders,* not *below the waist.*

Given that women's sexual desire starts in the brain, it's not surprising that hypoactive sexual desire disorder (HSDD)—which refers to the absence of sexual desire—is not only the most common form of female sexual dysfunction, it is also one of the most complicated, most undetected, under discussed, and untreated! For the *one third of the female population* that suffer from HSDD, factors may vary, but the frustration and pain of those factors form a common thread. And, unlike the fact that there are *twenty-six* approved medications for male erectile dysfunction, there are *two* for women—by the way, the one FDA-approved medication for HSDD is approved for women to use in *pre-menopause*, leaving all menopausal women with very few treatment options. That said, I hope to bring awareness to what I refer to as **The Collapsed V**.

A patient case in point:

> *Laura B., a vital (menopausal) fifty-five-year-old clothing designer and stylist, jets all over the globe for her international clients. No one could even begin to guess her correct age just by looking at her, and I defy anyone to believe that she is in menopause. But the fact is, despite a loving relationship with her husband of many years, Laura came to me after four months of avoiding intercourse. Aside from extreme vaginal dryness, she had been experiencing vaginal swelling and symptoms of a bladder infection after sex. She would feel the urgency to pee and a pressure upon urination. We ruled out infection, and then, a week later, after having intercourse for the first time in four months, an exam revealed that her visibly irritated vagina had evidence of superficial tearing. She said to me, "I feel like I'm losing my virginity every time I have sex now!"*

I coined **The Collapsed V** in order to classify a problem that I see every day in my practice, a problem that the medical world has been slow to acknowledge and slower still to address with any real solutions.

For women in menopause, the most common complaint (cry) I hear is dryness in the vagina. Unfortunately, dryness isn't just a problem for menopausal women; it affects women with breast cancer and those who are undergoing treatment for other types of cancer as well as women who have infrequent vaginal intercourse. As a matter of fact, a thirty-four-year-old patient of mine—because of her husband's chronic illness and inability to have an erection without a little blue pill—only has sex a few times a year. And, even though her relationship with her husband has been emotionally satisfying (and they've been creative in their physical connection), her vagina has suffered from "inactivity." She, too, has what I refer to as a **Collapsed V**.

Despite the fact that you may feel comfortable talking to your OB-GYN or your girlfriends about sex, you may hesitate to bring up your dehydrated or inactive vagina. But you ought not suffer in silence. The Collapsed V is a problem that is all too common, one that we need to talk about and find solutions for, if we are to experience sexual intimacy beyond menopause or illness or infrequent romantic encounters. First, it's important to figure out the cause of your Collapsed V, which, in many cases, has to do with the "M" word.

## Menopause

Ah, yes, menopause—the great equalizer of women. Finally accepted your AARP card? Congrats. But what might be even more helpful than discounted movie tickets is a better understanding of the sobering statistics of menopause and how it affects your vagina:

* Menopause makes everything on your body dry—your eyes, hair, mouth, skin, and especially your vagina. The vagina also becomes more narrow, shorter, less flexible, and smaller at the opening.
* There are 64 million postmenopausal women in the US, of which at least 50 percent suffer from vulvovaginal

atrophy, now known as Genitourinary Syndrome of Menopause (GSM).

* GSM is under-diagnosed and undertreated.
* The two most common symptoms of GSM include pain with sexual penetration and vaginal dryness.
* Painful intercourse—medically known as dyspareunia—is not covered by insurance. Absurdly enough, while erectile dysfunction is considered by insurance companies to be a medical condition, dyspareunia is considered a "lifestyle issue," and therefore, is not covered by most medical insurance.
* Only 7 percent of women are taking prescription medication to treat GSM.
* Out-of-pocket costs, lack of symptom improvement, and concerns about long-term estrogen exposure of the estrogen medication frequently prescribed for GSM, discourage women from being consistent with treatment.
* Estrogen patches—often used as treatment for GSM—may cost as much as $150, whereas testosterone patch treatment for men usually runs around two dollars.
* "Health care providers do not pay attention to midlife sexuality or female sexuality in general," states Dr. Sheryl Kingsberg, president of the North American Menopause Society (NAMS).
* Women are not being educated that their GSM symptoms are related to menopause.

Treatment for GSM must include ways to make the vagina less dry and the vaginal opening less narrow. Initially, doctors need to be doing a much better job of discussing the symptoms of GSM with their patients and how it may impact their sexual relationships.

The bottom line is that menopause can be f%$*ing brutal on the vagina. With your new normal of hot flashes and weight gain, irritability, mood swings, heart palpitations, and insomnia, it seems unfair that you would also have to deal with a new state of your vagina, especially since vaginal dryness becomes most apparent *after* you've begun to weather all the other effects of menopause. If you've opted out of any type of estrogen therapy, vaginal dryness usually becomes most disruptive around the fourth or fifth year after the onset of menopause, which means that any type of vaginal penetration, either with a penis, fingers, vibrator, or dildo may cause pain. However, your vagina does not have to give in to the hormonal disadvantages that come with menopause and a lack of estrogen. There *are* ways to help the vagina to retain its elasticity and pliability in order to avoid pain and discomfort with sex.

## Breast and Other Female Cancers

Many women become fixated on the statistic of "one in eight women are diagnosed with cancer." For many, the question isn't "if"—it's "when" will I contract that disease? For the majority of those women who are diagnosed with breast or other female cancers, sexual dysfunction will go hand in hand with a diagnosis.

Since estrogen is often an enemy to breast and other female cancers, part of a treatment plan may involve medications to stop estrogen production, which sets the stage for worsening vaginal dryness and a decreased interest in sex all together. Although it stands to reason that sex may not be high on a list of "to dos" for a woman battling cancer, physical intimacy can play an important part in maintaining one's sense of self. Unfortunately, and all too often, a woman who misses her sexual self may feel uncomfortable or selfish in discussing that particular loss, especially with the oncologist who is trying to save her life. For her, sexual intimacy becomes the elephant in the room.

The oncologist who sees his or her patient weekly may rarely bring up the topic of intimacy and sex, and therein lies part of the problem. No one is comfortable talking about sexual dysfunction as a byproduct of illness. In fact, The Lance Armstrong Foundation found that only 13 percent of women going through cancer treatment discussed their sexual dysfunction with their health care provider. Ideally, cancer treatment should involve someone with the proper training in sexual dysfunction—a psychologist or a sex therapist—that can deal with a patient's sexual health. As I discussed further in the **Pink V** chapter in my first book, there are many landmines women suffering from breast and other female cancers experience as they embrace their role as cancer survivor—or cancer thriver.

Cancer can be a triple whammy as it is also accompanied by the loss of sexual intimacy and sexual penetration with one's partner—all ingredients for a Collapsing V.

## Infrequent Sexual Penetration

Literally, "if you don't use it, you'll lose it!" Over time, with disuse—meaning that you don't use your vagina for sexual pleasure—your vaginal opening will become smaller and smaller. Now, of course, it will never close up completely, but shrinkage or collapse will occur. Eventually, you may completely disassociate or divorce yourself from your vagina altogether. You may talk yourself into believing you really don't want to have sex or penetration, or you may find yourself saying, "Cuddling is all that matters for a woman my age." Well, the woman who said that to me was only sixty-two. Frankly, I was surprised that she'd given up on her vagina and her desire to enjoy sex with her longtime partner.

If you take into consideration that the average life span for a woman is around *eighty years*, sixty-two seems awfully early to be retiring your vagina. Don't you think?

In fact, as long as we're talking "retirement," I feel like I ought to bring up the vagina that has been in perpetual retirement, and by that I mean the "virgin" vagina, a vagina that has never been penetrated with a penis or dildo. First off, I'd like to say: *It's never too late.* And if you are starting late, or starting early, or coming out of "retirement," please consider a vaginal dilator, as it will definitely make a world of difference.

When you have sexual intercourse for the first time (or you're penetrating your vagina with a dildo or even a finger for the first time) it is common and completely normal to experience some degree of pain, discomfort, and bleeding, which is why using a vaginal dilator is a good way of readying yourself. I don't know any "first timer" who hasn't thought, "How much pain will I experience my first time?" or "When will I stop bleeding?" or "How long will it take for sex to actually feel good?" To that end, I've always wondered, "Who decided that this "first time" female rite of passage should involve so much pain?"

Even the term "popping the cherry" sounds daunting. For starters, it can be helpful to understand that this term refers to the breaking of a woman's hymenal ring, the thin, circular or crescent shaped fold of mucous membrane over the vaginal opening, which varies in shape and size from woman to woman. This hymenal ring is the "cherry," and although it is broken with sexual intercourse, it can also break with recurrent tampon use, exercise, masturbation, or fingers. In other words, you can be the first to pop your own cherry, if you so desire!

## Vaginismus

As discussed in the TLC V chapter, Vaginismus is a condition in which the muscles of the vagina contract, tighten, or spasm involuntarily, causing vaginal pain, sexual discomfort, burning, and penetration problems. One commonly experiences symptoms on an ongoing basis—during sexual intercourse, inserting a tampon, and during a pelvic examination—resulting in a disruption of intimacy, personal relationships, and daily life activities. Vaginismus is both emotionally challenging and physically painful, especially when even the most basic of habits, such as tampon use is cause for anxiety and fear. It has ruined relationships and self-esteem, and claimed responsibility for sexless, unconsummated marriages.

But there is no longer a reason for any woman to suffer in silence from a Collapsed V caused by this condition or any other, for that matter. There are better ways!

## Clitoris: Out of Service

Unfortunately, the collateral damage of a Collapsing V can often include what I would describe as an "out of service" clitoris—medically referred to as acquired orgasmic dysfunction (AOD).

If you're finding it harder and harder to have an orgasm in menopause, it may be because your clitoris is no longer taking the hint. Physiologically, it makes sense, especially when you consider how helpful estrogen is in achieving orgasm. When the ovaries stop producing estrogen, this translates in less blood flow to the vulva, clitoris, and vagina, causing the entire area to become thinner, drier, and more delicate. A combination of menopause and other medical conditions such as diabetes and side effects of certain medications makes having an orgasm that much harder, if not impossible.

## Treatment for the Collapsing V

It took months, if not years, for your vagina to join the ranks of Collapsed V, so, in order to restore it, to make it vital and elastic again, you must dedicate yourself to new routines and habits that may take anywhere from a few weeks to a few months in order to see results. You must embrace a new normal in *feminine rituals.* These new routines may feel as welcome as calculus homework, at first, but your Collapsing V will ultimately benefit from those treatment routines—which may include hydration/moisturizing, dilation, physical therapy, and HRT (hormone replacement therapy), or some combination thereof.

### *Hydration, Please!*

First order in avoiding pain in vaginal penetration is to begin with a moist vagina.

You may remember a time when just the thought of intimacy and sex made you "wet." Imagination and anticipation may have been all you needed, and it may have worked great in your twenties and thirties, but, with life and all the complications that come with growing older, getting wet is probably not as easy as it used to be.

Chances are that, if you're nearing (or over) fifty, unless you have the proper foreplay to become sexually aroused, "getting wet" may, sadly, be impossible. If the vagina does not get wet, it means that it isn't producing a natural lubricant, the result of which is dry, painful vaginal sex. Also, the friction of sexual contact and penetration can cause the natural vaginal lubricants to dry up. Ultimately, this may be due to a drop in estrogen, caused by—you guessed it—menopause.

In fact, the two main hormonal assaults on the body that result in a drop in estrogen—and lead to a dry vagina—are menopause and breastfeeding. Of course, breastfeeding occurs during your *reproductive years,* while menopause typically happens at around age fifty. But the good news is that both of these hormonal conditions leading to vaginal dryness are reversible. Once you stop breastfeeding, the vagina will return to its normal healthy and hydrated state. However, dryness in menopause may be remedied with a variety of treatments, including vaginal estrogen, DHEA, hyaluronic acid, HRT, over-the-counter lubricants, vaginal suppositories, and laser treatment.

Additionally, the Mona Lisa Laser treatment—a treatment similar to facial micro-abrasion in that it removes dead cells and increases blood flow and collagen production *inside the vagina*—has been proven successful in battling dryness. Three painless three-minute sessions just six weeks apart and yearly thereafter seem to do the trick. In between treatments, vFit, a home-use intimate wellness device using red light therapy, can help to promote blood flow and natural vaginal lubrication by improving pelvic floor tissue and muscles. Together,

Mona Lisa and vFit make a great team in combatting vaginal dryness and getting your vagina back into shape! For those not ready for Mona Lisa, vFit is a great start.

### *Dilators to the Rescue!*

Also referred to as expanders, dilators should be part of any conversation with your health care provider in combating a Collapsed V. Relatively new in the arsenal to battle vaginal dryness, dilators have been lauded as a welcome and effective treatment as they can re-train, expand, and gently stretch the entrance and canal of the vagina.

If you're trying this method, it's recommended to use a *set* of vaginal dilators varying in sizes and thickness, from small to large—soft silicone dilators are the most comfortable and work best with the vagina as they minimize vaginal infections and tearing. The trick is to start with the smallest size and leave it inside the vagina for five to twenty minutes, two to four times a week. Duration of therapy is individualized for each woman, depending on the cause and circumstances of dryness. Best to use a comfortable lubricant or extra virgin coconut oil as you insert the dilator while lying on your back with your knees bent. In fact, a well-lubricated dilator and vagina is a must! Performing Kegel exercises at the same time as insertion is thought to help relax the pelvic floor muscles and make the process easier.

Your gynecologist can show you how to use your dilators correctly, but it is up to you to control the frequency of use and the speed in which you advance to larger-sized dilators. Relaxation exercises and physical therapy can also play an important part in dilator therapy, helping to make the process a success.

Up until now, dilators were designed for use only while lying down. Unfortunately, that did not bear well for the multi-tasking women of today who need to do the dishes or read bedtime stories to their kids while doing dilator therapy. With that in mind, I designed wearable dilators to be used while standing and multi-tasking. (No, I haven't thought of *everything,* but I'm trying.)

Since the biggest problem with effective dilator treatment has always been poor compliance, I'm hoping women will turn to this new and improved model to help themselves.

## *PT (Physical Therapy) for the Vagina*

As easy as it is to relate to PT for back or knee pain, PT for the vagina and bladder may sound a bit foreign to most women, but it turns out that PT for pelvic issues is growing in acceptance and popularity as a last resort in resolving issues related to painful sex and bladder dysfunction.

In fact, there are physical therapists trained in exactly this field. These qualified therapists will meet with you in order to get a clear understanding of the nature of your symptoms and then follow up with a pelvic exam in order to identify areas of weakness in and around the vagina. The therapy itself usually involves weekly sessions of stretching and massaging the outer and inner vagina in order to treat the areas of discomfort. I designed the first of it's kind She-ology wearable dilators to be used while standing and multi-tasking to stretch the vaginal opening, restore vaginal capacity by expanding the vagina in width and depth, and help users resume comfortable and more enjoyable sexual intercourse or self-stimulation.

As with any other health professionals, you may get a referral for a vaginal physical therapist from a trusted health care provider or from your gynecologist. You may even find that your gynecologist is trained in just this sort of therapy. You won't know until you ask.

### *Hormone Replacement Therapy (HRT)*

There has been a decided rush to judgment in recent years as to whether or not HRT is helpful or hurtful in the long run. In fact, the landmark Women's Health Initiative Study (WHI) in 2002, which examined hormone replacement therapy (HRT) and its impact on breast cancer, heart disease, and osteoporosis has been the biggest deterrent to women considering estrogen replacement therapy. The study's conclusions caused enough panic among women so that HRT became a dirty word. Truth is that the findings were inconclusive in many ways, as results varied depending upon the health of individual women. Subsequently, it was concluded, "Hormone therapy affects many organ systems in the body and changes the risks of many diseases—some in good ways, others in bad ways. Depending on hysterectomy status, age, and other individual factors, the consequences can vary dramatically."

What is now understood is that HRT is safe for many women to use within the ten-year period of time from the onset of menopause. The bottom line is that menopausal women need personalized care in their treatment, not information from generalized studies. Their vaginas depend on it!

### *Vibrators: Still a Girl's Best Friend*

In addition to the varied treatments for a dry vagina (or out-of-commission clitoris), I always suggest trying a vibrator. Especially in the case of acquired orgasmic dysfunction (AOD), which I talked about earlier, a vibrator can be an easy solution in helping to achieve orgasm when the aging process seems like it's arm wrestling you in the bedroom.

I would love to normalize the conversation about the usefulness of vibrators in treating orgasmic dysfunction. Not only do orgasms ease the stress of everyday living, they also work out the pelvic floor—which helps with incontinence. In addition, they are good for the heart, the mind, and the soul.

Do yourself a favor and give yourself the gift of my favorite vibrator, the Inspire Vibrating Ultimate Wand by Caloxotics. (Amazon Prime can get it to your nightstand by tomorrow morning!)

The unfortunate fact is that many women will suffer from painful sex for years before broaching the subject with a health care provider. It's been reported that "30 percent of women experience pain with vaginal sex and most don't tell their partners when sex hurts." Don't wait, please. Aside from the common issues I've mentioned, there are many other diagnosable and treatable causes of a vagina that feels like it's collapsing under pain! Those causes include:

* **Vaginal Infection.** The signs and symptoms of a vaginal infection may include vaginal discharge, odor, or itching, which may be the cause of your vaginal pain and swelling with sex. A trip to your health care provider will keep you educated.
* **Pelvic Inflammatory Disease (PID).** Sexually transmitted infections (STIs) such as Chlamydia and Gonorrhea are the typical culprits of PID, a serious pelvic infection that can lead to infertility and pelvic

pain. Getting STI checkups is especially important when you change sexual partners.

* **Penis Size.** "Bigger is better" is not the case for a vagina that can't tolerate a long, thick penis. The average penis is 5.7 inches in length and 4.8 inches in diameter (girth). When flaccid (not erect) the average penis measures between three and five inches. When erect, the average penis measures between five and seven inches. The vagina may stretch to accommodate a larger sized penis, but it may take time, patience, strategic sexual positions, vaginal dilators, and open communication.
* **Vaginal Tears and Lacerations.** Tears and lacerations can result from many things—sex without proper lubricant, a larger-than-average penis, use of a particular sex toy, or trauma from childbirth. Vaginal lubricants can help avoid some of these problems.
* **Latex Allergy.** The majority of condoms are made out of latex, which propose little problem to most women, except those with latex allergies. An allergic reaction to latex may involve vaginal swelling, itching, and pain during and up to thirty-six hours after sex. If you have a latex allergy, you can use a polyurethane condom as an alternative for your safe sex measures.
* **Ruptured Ovarian Cyst.** If you are having sex during ovulation or mid-cycle, chances are there is an expected large ovarian cyst waiting to ovulate and release the egg. Aggressive sex can cause this cyst to rupture, releasing its fluid contents along with the egg and causing pain. A pelvic ultrasound combined with your menstrual history can help with a proper diagnosis.

* **Endometriosis and Uterine Fibroids.** Both of these female problems can cause pain with sex, especially with deep penetration. A detailed health history, pelvic ultrasound, and a discussion with your health care provider of other related symptoms are necessary in order to detect these conditions.
* **Positional Sex.** Certain sexual positions are known to be anatomically hard on the vagina and female organs, including the uterus and ovaries. The missionary position tends to be anatomically easier for women, whereas Doggie Style or "from behind," which allows for deeper penetration for the male, may bring more discomfort and pain for many women.
* **Virginal.** If you have never had vaginal penetration with a penis, your first experience with sex will probably be painful. It may take time and regular sex before you start to experience anything like pleasure. Prepping the hymenal ring with a vaginal dilator a month before penetration would be a novel and effective plan. Also, a good lubricant or numbing gel (lidocaine) at the entrance of the vagina can also help relieve pain. In any case, patience and good communication with your partner is the right recipe for success.
* **Emotional Problems.** Depression, anxiety, relationship problems, and fear of intimacy all play a role in painful sex. Psychotherapy and the ability to communicate your feelings to your partner can help overcome some of the emotional problems that may inhibit a healthy, enjoyable sex life.
* **History of Sexual Abuse.** Any history of sexual abuse and trauma (emotional or physical) can contribute to

> an aversion or general dislike of sex. A devastating experience that leads to "post-traumatic stress disorder" may only enable you to feel pain with sex. As in dealing with emotional problems, therapy and open communication with your partner is key to helping resolve issues linked to abuse and trauma.

When it comes to dealing with the cause, effect, and treatment of a Collapsed V, women simply want the same responsiveness from the medical community as men have had with their sexual issues.

Think about this: A man walks into his doctor's office with a complaint about his inability to have or maintain an erection, and then he walks out with a little blue pill. Boom. A woman walks into the same doctor's office with a complaint of period pain and pain with sex. If the underlying cause of that pain is endometriosis, it will take, on average, *9.2 years* for that woman to be correctly diagnosed, as reported in Lili Loofbourow's illuminating 2018 essay, "The female price of male pleasure."

In that same essay, Loofbourow noted that *PubMed* (the database for the National Center for Biotechnology Information) has 393 clinical trials studying female dyspareunia—the severe physical pain experienced during sex—10 clinical trials studying vaginismus, 43 studying vulvodynia, and 1,954 devoted to the study of erectile dysfunction. Here's the math: There are five times as many clinical trials on male sexual pleasure as on female sexual pain. Women are the ones who forego the conversation on their own sexual health and experiences, since society seems to be telling them that the ultimate goal of the sexual experience is a man's orgasm. That is not an ultimate goal. The goal needs to be an equally shared and equally satisfying experience, one that is *pain-free*.

It is time for women not to feel shame or embarrassment about issues of their own sexual dysfunction. In fact, the FDA is finally showing support for the challenges faced in female sexual health by researching and approving viable new treatment options. There *are* health providers out there who are willing to listen and act, and there are treatment options available—even if they don't come in the form of an easy-to-swallow, *little blue pill*. As women, our needs are a bit more complicated than that—to which I say, "Amen."

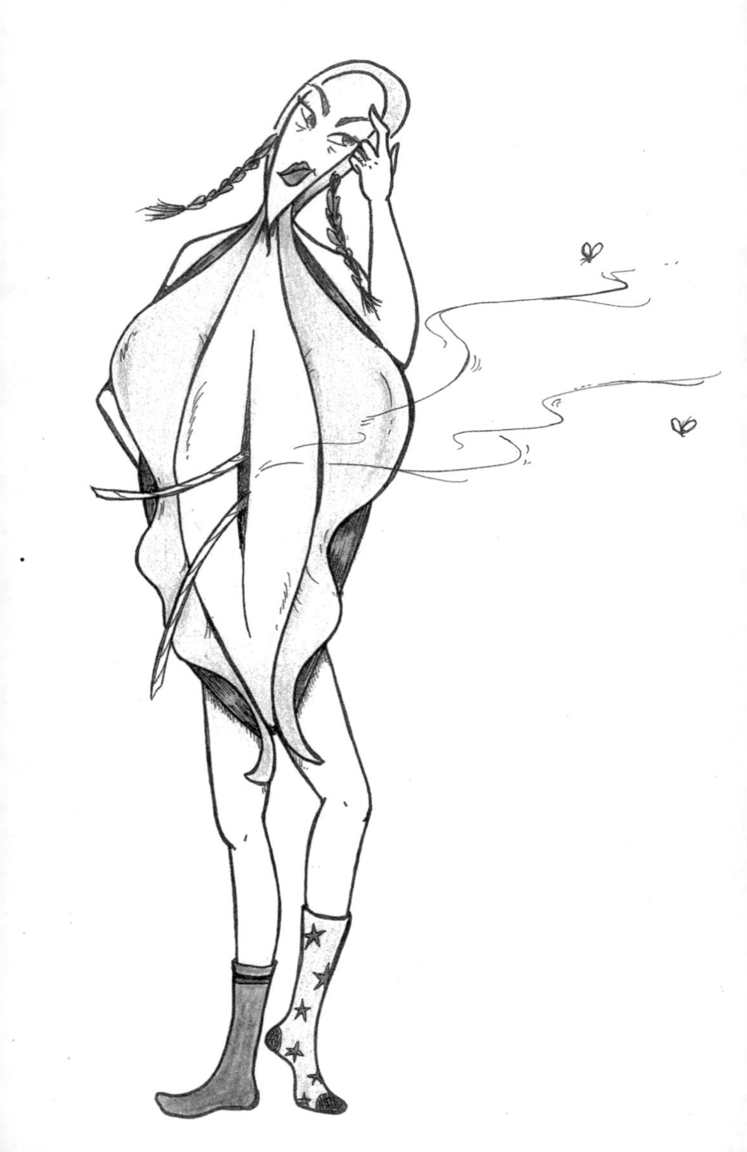

# CHAPTER 12

# forgetful

"Twenty years after the fact, the mere thought of that 'forgotten' tampon still terrifies me. I remember the moment like it was yesterday: 9 p.m. on a school night; I was a seventeen-year-old in a panic, calling my forever OB-GYN, Dr. Sherry, way after hours (I wonder if she ever regretted giving me her cell phone number). I don't even recall if I said hello before blurting out, 'I know I left a tampon in my vag and I have to see you!'

Dr. Sherry could tell I was not going to take 'come to my office in the morning' as an answer because I was sure I'd be dead from Toxic Shock Syndrome by then, so she told me to come to her house for a special visit—it was only later I found out that it wasn't unusual for her to have patients over for these 'reverse' house calls. When I arrived at 10 p.m., apparently horror-stricken, she was calm and reassuring, as she showed me to the empty bedroom of her fourteen-year-old son, Michael, where I had to undress from the waist down. She handed me a beach towel, and, as professional as she was, I suddenly found it hilarious to be surrounded by posters of Pikachu, Mandy Moore, and Star Wars! Equipped with her usual sterile speculum and gloves—with the added help of a household flashlight—Dr. Sherry rolled a computer chair closer to me. As I scooched to the edge of her son's bed, my legs spread eagle in the air—Mandy and Darth Vader looking down on me from opposite walls—I swore to myself: This will *never* happen again.

Those three minutes were the longest three minutes of my life, as I held my breath, praying that Dr. Sherry would come up empty from her scavenger hunt. Luckily, she didn't find any hidden tampons in the long and endless hiding place formerly known as my vagina.

My BFFs and I laugh about this story now, but I totally understand how this can happen even to the most conscientious of us women. Toxic Shock Syndrome is nothing to joke about, especially after learning from the Lauren Wasser story how quickly women can get it and how destructive it can become.

In Dr. Sherry's Forgetful V, she points out how hard it can sometimes be to keep track of tampons going in and tampons going out. My advice is definitely: When in doubt about a lost tampon, make an appointment with your doctor so you don't have to have the *unforgettable* experience that I had! ”

—**Sara Foster** Actress

## A Forgotten Tampon Gives New Meaning to the Term "Lost"

Have you ever wondered whether you've taken out the last tampon you put in? If the answer is an emphatic "yes," you might be relieved to know how often I treat what is medically called—get ready for it—"lost tampon." Certainly, it's at least testament to how often we multitask, causing us to forget certain basics such as our last tampon change.

*Tori, an energetic, fun-loving twenty-one-year-old college student could, admittedly, uncover a happy hour in a ghost town. Back at home recently on spring break, she and three of her Delta Gamma Sorority sisters had Ubered to their favorite Mexican restaurant in Manhattan Beach. After a few rounds of skinny margaritas, Tori returned home a bit tipsy and exhausted by a happy hour party that had extended to midnight. She figured that, at some point during her numerous bathroom runs, she'd pulled out her last tampon—she later recalled: "You know how sometimes you just don't see the string?"—so she stuck in a new one before going to bed. A couple weeks after her period ended, she noticed a foul smell coming from her vagina. She investigated with a finger and pulled out some brownish discharge that smelled (she said) "like I was standing on the edge of a fishing pier!" By the end of the day, she was up in stirrups in my exam room and I was reaching for the closest bio-hazardous bag I could find. In one quick motion, I pulled out the two-week-old tampon that had been deeply wedged up in Tori's vagina. As fast as my nurse Dani could secure the bag and run it down the hall, it wasn't fast enough to prevent the awful, no-tampon-should-stick-around-this-long stench that filled the office. Oops. Tori was mortified, but I just wanted to be sure that she didn't have a yeast or bacterial infection, or worse. She didn't.*

Not only are tampons "lost" more often than one would realize, the fact is that tampons can easily be pushed and turned sideways into the back of the vagina, hiding them from not-so-plain sight. Normally, a tampon runs along in a parallel direction inside the vagina. If a second tampon is accidently pushed inside the vagina, the original tampon can turn sideways, perpendicular to the end of the vagina, and the second one would completely obscure it.

In this case, you may start experiencing symptoms such as brown, gray, or green vaginal discharge, pungent odor, vaginal pain, and uterine cramping. If you experience unusual pain in inserting a tampon, it may suggest that you have a second tampon at the end of that vaginal tunnel. You can always do a self-check in the privacy of your own home to determine whether a sideways tampon is lodged up in wait. Also, it's a good excuse to really get to know your vagina. Here's what I would suggest: Wash your hands well, put one leg on the toilet seat cover, and with your pointer finger reach all the way into the back of your vagina. If you do, indeed, hit the jackpot and pull out one very smelly, old tampon, this would be the *one time* I would suggest following up with a simple water-vinegar douche.

If your search is in vain, but you still think that there's *something up there,* don't hesitate to contact your health care provider. Believe me, they have seen it all (and worse) and taking time out of your busy day to ensure your health might well turn out to be a *lifesaving* venture. If you're not feeling sick, it's more than likely that you are fine (lost tampon or not), but, on very rare occasions, something more may be brewing.

## Toxic Shock Syndrome

Fifteen-year-old Rylie Whitten thought she had the flu—strangely enough, accompanied by a sunburn-like rash. The Michigan teen made the health news headlines when her diagnosis came back as TSS (Toxic Shock Syndrome) as a result of tampon use, even though she hadn't left one in longer than *eight hours*. Rylie suffered kidney and other organ damage due to a highly absorbent tampon and was put on life support. Fortunately, she survived, but she and many others learned of what a lethal and random illness TSS is.

Lauren Wasser, a successful young model, also thought she had the flu during her period. She'd always been careful to change her tampons regularly, so, when she'd begun to feel sick after only a few hours of having changed her last tampon, the tampon was the last culprit she would have considered. By the time she headed home from a friend's house, she was too sick to do anything but pass out in bed. She felt even worse when she woke and decided to go back to sleep. That's the last thing she remembered. Lauren was found the following day on the bathroom floor, unconscious, with a fever of 107. She was rushed to the hospital with organ failure and suffered a heart attack. Lauren's life was saved, but at the cost of both her legs to TSS.

Lauren has since turned this devastating experience into one of inspiration. She continues to model with her prosthetic legs and feels that she's been given the opportunity to share a different vision of beauty, one that includes imperfection.

**Toxic Shock Syndrome** is an extremely rare, complicated bacterial infection caused by toxins produced by the Staph bacteria. From 1980 to 1989, there were sixty-one reported cases of TSS, although, over the last ten years, there have only been four cases reported annually. Statistically, TSS affects one in every 100,000 people, with half of those dying from this destructive infection. The syndrome is thought to occur only in menstruating women, but men, children, and postmenopausal women may also contract it, although about half the cases do occur in the former group, especially among women who use super-absorbent tampons. Those types of tampons can serve as a breeding ground for the Staph bacteria that ends up in the bloodstream, especially if they are left in for over eight hours. For the men, children, and postmenopausal women who contract TSS, the bacteria are introduced through surgical infections, burns, sinusitis, skin lesions, and postpartum wound infections, such as mastitis.

In women who have contracted TSS from tampon use, symptoms of TSS can occur quickly and without warning, typically between the second and fifth day of their menstrual cycle. As we've seen in the case of Rylie Whitten, TSS can start out as a fever and sunburn-like rash, especially on the hands and feet, along with vomiting, muscle aches, headaches, or diarrhea. The "sunburn" rash appearing on the palm of the hands and bottoms of the feet is the characteristic skin change of TSS. Symptoms may progress to lowered blood pressure, ulcerations in mucous membranes such as eyes, mouth, and throat, ultimately causing difficulty in breathing, and, in many cases, death.

Testing for TSS can be difficult. First and foremost, a thorough physical exam along with the review of a patient's medical history is vital in establishing a correct diagnosis. Vaginal cultures of the vagina and cervix along with blood and urine samples to check for Staph or Strep infections are part of the process. If any cultures prove positive, or you develop symptoms of TSS, antibiotic treatment is prescribed, and, depending on the severity, hospitalization may be necessary.

Best prevention? Tampons should be changed *every two to six hours*, and never—I mean, *never*—leave a tampon in for more than eight hours. Using a low absorbency tampon will also minimize risk. Many health care professionals suggest alternating tampons with sanitary pads whenever possible, especially if your blood flow is very light. If you are a fan of the menstrual cup, never leave it in place for more than twelve hours. Adopting a routine of regularly changing your tampons will not only help prevent unwanted odors and infections, it can help prevent the more lethal TSS.

Yes, TSS is rare but, when it happens, it can be life threatening. I say this to educate you of the need not to panic about this toxic syndrome. Take the simple precautions mentioned here and know the signs and symptoms associated with this disease, which, if recognized quickly, can be treated. If you are on your period or have recently finished it and you notice any of the symptoms discussed here, call your doctor immediately.

Talk about *forgetful*! Forget your keys, forget an appointment or lunch, even forget your partner's birthday; it's nothing compared to the possible physical harm of forgetting what you've put in your vagina. Better to be plain embarrassed by your forgetful V, rather than terrified by it. Don't forget!

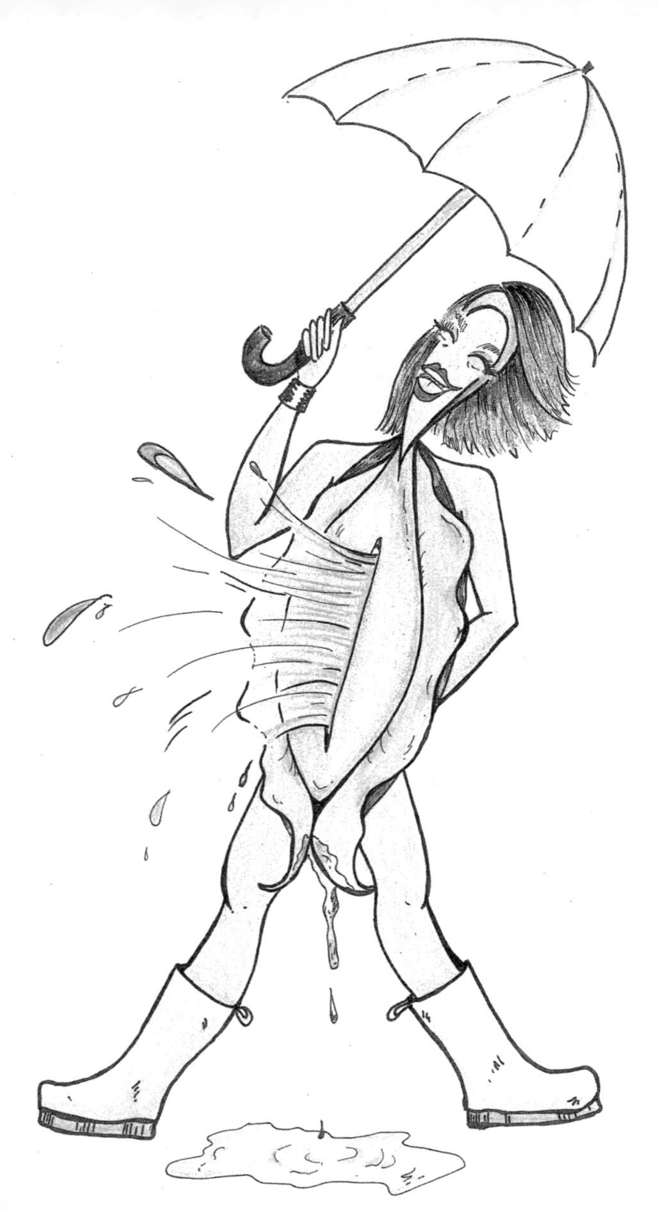

CHAPTER 13

# squirting

"Before Dr. Sherry asked me to comment on 'squirting'—a.k.a. female ejaculation—I thought it was this magical, amazing thing women occasionally did during orgasm. I mean, it's what I do. I figured it was a given, that is, before I asked around and then Googled it. Imagine my surprise when I pulled up, like, a million articles pointing to 'the squirt' as this presumed Mount Everest of G-spot stimulation, and I realized the pressure some women felt in trying to 'achieve' it. Really? An achievement? You mean like flat abs and hair-free bodies? Yeah, the hair-free thing, that's disturbing as well—I mean, I love sex as much as the next person, but, because I've been monogamous for so long, I didn't realize that not only are you not allowed to have any hair 'down there,' but, when you hit the highest high of orgasm, you need to gush like a popped juice box [horrible visual intended]. What happened to just trying not to wake your neighbors?

The very first time I squirted during sex was also one of the first times I had lesbian girl sex. Since I never gushed with a man, I assumed it was something that women did with other women. I believed that male and female fingers were so different that only girls could make me go off like a sprinkler. Now I'm finding out that, apparently, hetero women and their partners are under the gun. Listen, heterosexuals everywhere, I'm brokenhearted that you have one more thing on your sexual 'must do' list. Trust me, it's just going to make you more neurotic and disappointed than you deserve to be.

My advice? Embrace the squirt if it's in your sexual DNA—never be embarrassed by it—but, more importantly, don't sweat it if ye old G-spot ain't the water pistol that your latest, favorite gal magazine tells you it should be. ”

—**Suzanne Westenhoefer** Comedian

## Squirting: What's Going On?!

I've been asked this question many ways, some of which are:

Is it normal to "squirt?"

Am I having, like, the Super Bowl experience of sex?

Is *gushing* an urban legend?

Okay, so no one *really* knows the exact statistics about who can squirt or who actually does squirt, so, with that uncertainty in mind, it was found that 10 to 50 percent of women have, at one time or another, had a "gushing" moment during orgasm. In fact, a recent study presented in the December 2017 Journal of Sexual Medicine found that almost 70 percent of women ejaculate during orgasm—honestly, a staggering statistic by any standards.

## Squirting V

*Twenty-four-year-old Keisha was in grad school by night and supporting herself as a model by day. She'd never had reason to visit my office other than to have her yearly Pap smears, until she called for an appointment to discuss a certain "crazy thing" her body was doing during sex with her new boyfriend. "It's going to sound weird," she said. "But, sometimes during sex, I feel this gush and the bed gets soaked. At first, I thought I'd peed, but it's happening regularly now and I don't think that's it. What's going on?!" Keisha was sure she had a UTI or vaginal infection.*

In short, call it what you want—gushing, squirting, ejaculating—but what Keisha described to me is a true and real sexual phenomenon. Sometimes when women are sexually aroused or stimulated there is an expulsion of fluid from the glands around the urethra during or before orgasm. However, the fluid from this orgasmic expression is not coming from the vagina, but rather from the urethra. Although this expulsion of fluid can be related to G-spot stimulation, it's possible to squirt or gush without stimulation of the sexual sweet spot. Some women have reported squirting after giving blowjobs or having their nipples sucked.

You've heard the saying, haven't you? *Different strokes for different folks.* Gives that expression new meaning, doesn't it?

For some, like Keisha, the experience is likened to wetting the bed. For others is it less obvious. If you haven't heard about "the squirt" you may feel embarrassment in thinking that you *have* peed. If, indeed, the fluid is only composed of urine, you would need to discuss this with your healthcare provider, but you'll know if you've *gushed* because the liquid tastes and smells the same as the "wet" from orgasm. The fluid may contain *some* urine, but that's to be expected, since it's coming out of the urethra, which is the exit of the bladder.

> *I love my conversations with twenty-nine-year-old Sandy. One of my more sexually and socially liberal patients, she never has any qualms about expressing the details of what she deems her most life-changing experiences. During her recent Pap smear, she could hardly wait to share that she'd become a "bona fide squirter!" Seems Sandy's new girlfriend was quite talented in locating Sandy's G-spot right off the start, which, apparently, was a near-religious experience. She told me, "The orgasm builds up slowly and then I'm overtaken by waves of warmth going through my body as it builds. I have to allow myself to just go with it and not hold back in any way, physically or mentally. I'll be thinking that I want to continue because it feels so amazing, but yet it's also frightening because of the intensity, which, in the past, has made me want to stop. Like, I can feel so frantic because the feeling is so intense. But I finally allowed myself to just go with it and not hold back in any way, and then it happened! The gush, the whole thing, it was indescribable!"*

Embrace it, love it, and certainly don't shy away from this phenomenon if it's in the cards for you. This isn't to say that these particular "flowing" orgasms are somehow better or more intense than non-squirting, less juicy orgasms. They're just different, as different as the women who report them.

When women are sexually aroused, which often happens with stimulation of the G-spot, there usually is some degree of wetness in the vagina, which is an appropriate sexual response. Whether your orgasm is obvious or more subtle,

I say lucky you for having one! Either way, it's a satisfying experience.

## In Search of the G-Spot

There is an ongoing debate as to whether the G-spot—also known as the "sweet spot"—actually exists. Its exact location is a bit of a mystery, but there are different theories as to its existence. For those "believers," myself included, the G-spot is located one to three inches on the top or anterior surface of the vagina. If you insert your finger into the top surface of your vagina, up to about the second knuckle, the slightly bumpy mound or ridged area you reach can be identified as the G-spot (some describe it as having the same texture as a raisin). When a woman is sexually aroused, the G-spot fills with blood, giving it a swollen feeling. When properly stimulated, you may orgasm or even ejaculate!

Truth is that not all women respond sexually to stimulation of this apparently magical place known as the G-spot, so don't worry if you've tried and failed to locate it. It is not a magic button but, rather, another avenue in achieving sexual pleasure. If you haven't tried to locate it, you might want to try to do so, on your own or with your partner. That said, here are a few guidelines:

* First off, get in the right mood, alone or with your partner. Best to have no distractions and to feel relaxed. A gentle massage is a great starter and an enjoyable way to warm up. If you need a little extra lubricant, extra virgin coconut oil is a definite crowd pleaser.
* Insert your 2nd (index finger) and 3rd finger into your (or your partner's) well-lubricated vagina up to the

second knuckle. If you curve you finger(s) upward, you should be able to find the slightly bumpy mound or ridged area. Use a "come here" motion of your index finger. The texture of this area is unlike any other area in the vagina. You can start first with your 2nd finger, and then, as the vagina relaxes and opens, you can insert a 2nd finger.

* Your well-lubricated fingers should gently, at first, stroke the anterior surface of the upper vagina. Applying continuous pressure in this area may also give you the urge to pee, since you are having your urethra pressed, so be sure to empty your bladder before you start.
* When you're close to orgasm you may "push out" in the pelvic area, which can help you achieve a female ejaculation. (Very important: Make sure your fingernails are cut so that the delicate vaginal tissue isn't injured. Also, be sure that you or your partner is not suffering from any vaginal odor or itching, as this can definitely interfere with this exploration.)

It may take some time and practice in your search for the elusive G, so patience is truly a virtue, but the rewards are well worth your efforts!

As with "squirting," I am often asked about whether the G-spot itself is myth or phenomenon, and I can honestly say (from personal experience) that I know it exists. I'm glad when women feel open enough to ask about their own G-spots.

I heartily encourage you to try to find your G-spot, if you haven't already. It may be the "indescribable" experience that Sonia detailed, or it may be something else entirely. What is important in your exploration is to embrace your sexuality and get in sync with what makes you feel good in bed. If you know that you like, then you can more easily guide your partner—a win-win situation for you both.

Don't be embarrassed about your curiosity. Even at this stage of the game, my girlfriends and I will have a conversation over a pitcher of margaritas about who does and who doesn't squirt and about where everyone believes their G-spot to be. I've been known to draw diagrams on dinner napkins in order to illustrate "location." Have fun. Look for your G-spot. Love your squirting vagina. Even though it may not be easy (or practical) to be a regular "squirter," a squirting vagina knows how to purr!

"¡Ay Dios mío! Everyone had given up on me getting married. I was one of those women who really loved being single. I thought the only reason to get married was to have children. And, even though my biological clock became more like a ticking time bomb in my mid-thirties, I was still not ready, so I gave up on the whole idea of marriage *and* kids.

Then I met my prince—from Scotland, no less—in a totally random way at a bar in New York City. He had come to NYC for a first-time visit, and I was visiting my family after having moved to Los Angeles—where I had realized my dreams. I had my own national TV show, Kiki Desde Hollywood, and I was crossing over to Network TV with a development deal—I was about to be the Latina Oprah! Meeting the possible father of my children was not on my agenda.

But my V doesn't lie—that is, my *squirting V*. Okay, I'll explain. Maybe you saw Howard Stern interview a porn star who was a bona fide squirter, or maybe you heard Jenny McCarthy share the news that masturbating five times a day had made *her* a squirter—even if you thought, "Oh, Jenny, TMI, and, btw, please stop talking about not vaccinating your kids," or whatever—but that's what I mean. I always knew when I was interested in a man because I'd experience a squirting V. For me, it was a totally inexplicable sign of attraction.

My prince and I became great friends, at first. He was in the oil industry in Aberdeen, Scotland, and I was in the entertainment business in Hollywood. *How the heck would that relationship work?*

So we emailed. I told him my dating stories and he told me his. I even told him about a date I had with a TV executive where there was a mutual attraction, but, because I did not want to sleep my way to the top, I ignored my squirting V and ended up with a blue vagina!

No surprise: My Scottish bloke and I eventually married, and, after quite a bit of drama (which I'll save for Doctor Sherry's next book), we wound up with twins! So I've gotta give a little credit to my squirting V, which nudged me here in the first place. Although, I have to admit, as I get older—and having birthed two babies—I can no longer tell if my V is squirting out of attraction or because I desperately need a good, long pee. ”

—**Kiki Melendez** Actress and Producer

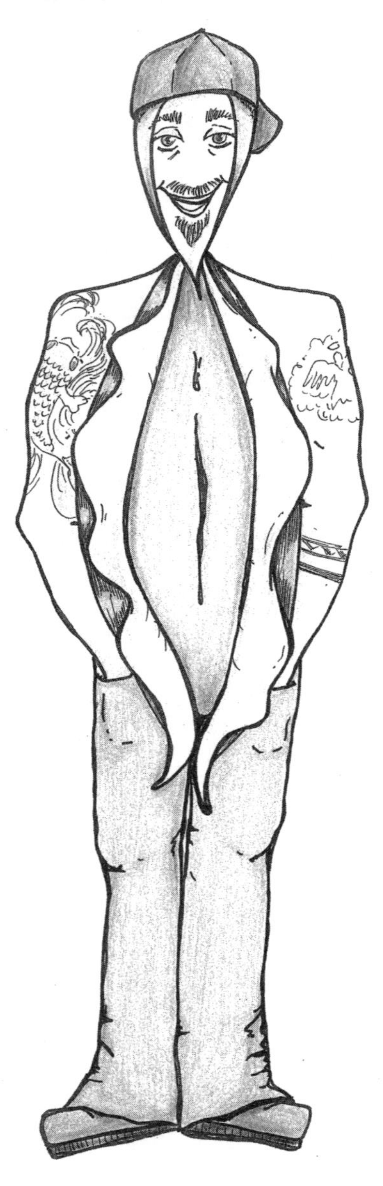

CHAPTER 14

# trans

Being transgender is not a choice, and it is not the anomaly that people once believed it to be. In fact, *2 to 5 percent* of the population is transgender. In the United States alone, nearly 150,000 young people and 1.4 million adults identify as transgender—an umbrella term for people whose gender identity and/or gender expression differs from what is typically associated with the sex they were assigned at birth. People under the transgender umbrella may describe themselves using one or more of a wide variety of terms.

Despite the number of people that identify as "trans," research on transgender people is limited and outdated, at best. The one fact that isn't outdated is that the trans people are at a higher risk for HIV/AIDS, addiction, and engagement in sex work. They face difficulty finding employment and maintaining consistent housing, and also experience high levels of violence. Most of these life challenges occur as a result of rejection and vilification due to the fact that they are transgender.

As far as the medical community's response to transgender people goes, most medical professionals don't have the necessary training to sensitively care for and address the needs of this particular group of people.

It is my aim to educate men and women on the transgender community through a medical lens and with an accepting heart. I have personally learned so much from my trans patients, so much so that I have asked them to partner with me here in order to help better serve them and their community, both medically and emotionally. Knowing and understanding a person's sexual identity is as important as knowing their names and opinions, likes and dislikes. We, as human beings, are one community with the same desires: to be respected, appreciated, heard, and loved—and to thrive in a safe and welcoming environment.

In order to understand the trans community and to have a concise and meaningful conversation about transgender people, it is important to at least begin by becoming familiar with the correct terminology, as it relates to them.

Sadly, though, doctors and other health care professions often do not have any greater understanding of this particular community than lay people—and often don't even know the correct terminology used in the trans population. As a health care provider, I have heard firsthand of how poorly trained most doctors and gynecologists are in treating female patients other than a straight cis woman.

Whether you are or aren't familiar with the term "cis woman," these definitions are for you. To begin with, let's be clear: "Gender identity is distinct from sexual orientation, sex development, and external gender expression."

* **Gender identity** refers to a person's innermost concept of self as male, female, a blend of both, or neither. One's gender identity can be the same or different from their sex assigned at birth.
* **Gender expression** is the external presentation of one's gender, as expressed through one's name, clothing, behavior, hairstyle, or voice, and which may or may not conform to socially defined behaviors and characteristics typically associated with being either masculine or feminine.
* **Gender diverse** is used to describe people who do not conform to their societal or cultural expectations for males and females. Being transgender is one way of being gender diverse, but not all gender diverse people are transgender.
* **Gender queer** refers to a person who is neither exclusively male nor female.
* **Assigned male at birth** refers to a person who was thought to be male when born and initially raised as a boy.
* **Assigned female at birth** refers to a person who was thought to be female at birth and initially raised as a girl.
* **Trans or transgender** is an umbrella term for someone whose gender identity is not congruent with their sex assigned at birth.
* **Cis gender** is a term for someone whose gender identity aligns with their sex assigned at birth.

* **Trans boy/male/man** is used to describe someone who was assigned female at birth who identifies as a boy/male/man.
* **Trans girl/female/woman** describes someone who was assigned male at birth who identifies as a girl/female/woman.
* **Non-binary** is a term to describe someone who doesn't identify exclusively as male or female.
* **Gender fluid** refers to a person whose gender identity varies over time.
* **Agender** is used to describe someone who does not identify with any gender.
* **Brotherboy and Sistergirl** are terms traditionally used by Aboriginal and Torres Strait Islander people in a number of different contexts, but often refer to trans and gender diverse people. Brotherboy typically refers to masculine spirited people who were assigned female at birth. Sistergirl typically refers to feminine spirited people who were assigned male at birth.
* **Gender dysphoria** is a term that describes the distress experienced by a person due to incongruence between their gender identity and their sex assigned at birth.
* **Social transition** is the process by which a person changes their gender expression to better match their gender identity.
* **Medical transition** is the process by which a person changes their physical sex characteristics via hormonal intervention and/or surgery to more closely align with their gender identity.

In referencing those who consider themselves transgender, one of several pronouns may be preferential, including he, she, they, and ze. Unfortunately, in writing, spell check seems not yet to have caught up with the times, especially when referring to a single person as "they." Like any relatively new reference, the dictionaries are the last to know!

As you can see, even though the term transgender may refer to 2 to 5 percent of the population, it is an umbrella term, certainly not a "one size fits all," in the same way that "woman" or "man" only *begins* to describe an individual. Also, such that a cis gender woman needs particular health care, so do women who were not born female, or men who *were* born female.

## Addressing the Basic Health Care Needs of Transgender People

Oliver, non-binary:

> *A little about me for context: I am a twenty-three-year-old Mexican American non-binary trans person who was assigned female at birth. I do not identify as a man, woman, male, female, etc. I consider my identity and my body void of gender, and my expression changes as I please. I also live with chronic pain, depression, and anxiety, but seeking care for all of these things has been difficult, due to a lack of transgender and queer competency in health care.*
>
> *Two particularly traumatizing experiences in the last two years deterred me from seeking that care. Two years ago, I moved to Philadelphia and went to a Planned Parenthood in Philly's Gayborhood (a predominantly gay and gay-friendly neighborhood in Philadelphia) thinking they would be competent in dealing with*

*transgender people. I had booked an appointment with a doctor to deal with my bacterial vaginosis. I had not legally changed my name (from my traditionally male Mexican name) so I tried to make it clear that my name was Oliver, not the name on my ID, and that I was non-binary. No one understood, so they didn't use my correct pronouns (they/them).*

*The female doctor said, "I haven't really worked with people like you." Then she examined my genitals, gendering my vulva as "she." I told her that made me uncomfortable and that it was inappropriate. Her response: "Honey, it doesn't matter what you are, SHE is always a SHE."*

*The doctor refused to respect my gender identity and insisted on using feminine pronouns for my body parts. I left crying.*

*A year and a half later, I went to the University of Pennsylvania's LGBT Medical Center in hopes of finding someone more competent to discuss my chronic back and knee pain. The forms asked for my preferred pronouns, which I gave, but they were ignored. At the time, I had just started hormones. I had been using testosterone gel for about two months and hesitated telling the doctor because I was afraid of what they would do or say, especially since I got the gel from a friend, not a doctor. Ultimately, I put my faith in the center and included the information. The doctor read my form and did not understand my gender identity, expression, or desire to be on hormones. She was a cis gender woman with a very narrow idea of what transgender meant. She was confused I did not identify as a man and that, although I was on testosterone, I did not want to be perceived as male. We had a fifteen-minute conversation about gender and hormones. She then got close to me, grabbed my arm and urged me to 'consider preserving my fertility.'*

*In fact, I have no desire to be pregnant or give birth, and I couldn't believe that a doctor would derail my appointment about my chronic pain to talk about something that I have thought long and hard about for years. I left the appointment in tears and stopped using testosterone in fear of interacting with more incompetent doctors."*

Dr. Tochi Iroku-Malize, MD, the chair of family medicine for Northwell Health, cares for many patients in the LGBTQIA (lesbian, gay, bisexual, transgender, queer, intersexual, or asexual) community and has stated, "People in this special population of patients may feel that the health care system, including providers and institutions, is not up to recognizing their culture or their needs."

Dr. Iroku-Malize has also pointed out that research shows "people who depart from traditional heterosexual norms feel disrespected and marginalized in health care settings. The literature also shows that these patients do in fact receive poorer quality care than people who fit prevailing norms." Obviously, the stigma against trans people is real and prevalent.

That stigma against trans people perpetuates their avoidance in going to doctors for basic care, depression, suicidal thoughts, substance abuse, and long-term medical conditions. It's not that physicians necessarily need to be experts in caring for trans patients, but they do need an awareness of this oft-neglected population and the *basics* of how to approach them.

For the most part, trans people are afraid that doctors and health care providers won't treat them as their gender identity selves, which is why it's imperative that doctors and office staff gain the trust of a trans patient before an initial exam. The first step toward gaining that trust is acknowledging how a trans person wants to be identified, and then having respect for that identification.

Clearly, the medical community needs to do more in extending an olive branch to this in-need population and understanding the health risks and barriers they commonly face.

Will, a trans male:

*I want to be transparent in saying that my experience is not going to be the same as many other transgender folks because I am cis-passing and often do not feel the need to disclose that I'm trans to doctors I won't be seeing long term. Last year, I had a hand injury that required I go to a specialist. Not knowing anything about the doctor, I didn't feel comfortable disclosing my trans status—besides, the health care was unrelated to my genitals. I did have to take off my shirt for some tests, but I had top surgery many years ago and have no scars, so I appeared "male." I didn't disclose that I'd had surgery or that I was on hormones for fear of mistreatment.*

*Instead, I'd say that 90 percent of my health care is done at my endocrinologist's office where they already know I'm trans. In fact, my most positive medical experiences have been at my endocrinologist's office—at the Beth Israel Medical Center in Manhattan. They see LGBTQ patients on a regular basis, so the first time I went there, they asked if my chosen name was different than my legal name and what pronouns I preferred. Because*

*I felt comfortable, I finally made an OB-GYN appointment at the center, something I'd been avoiding for years. The gynecologist happened to be a trans woman, so she understood how emotionally challenging the visit was. She took the time to talk me through the exam beforehand. I cannot imagine having a gynecological exam with someone I didn't know to be trans competent. Most trans people I know have been mis-gendered and disrespected at doctors' offices, when all they're trying to do is take care of their health. The myths of trans people weigh much heavier than the truths!*

## The Greatest Myths of Being Transgender

* Being transgender is a mental disorder.
* All transgender people want to transition with medication or top or bottom surgery.
* Transgender men and women are not real men and women.
* Sexual orientation is linked to gender identity.
* It's rude to ask how you should address someone.
* All trans people medically transition.
* Transitioning is as simple as one surgery.
* Children aren't old enough to know their gender identity.
* Transgender people are confused or are intent on confusing others.
* Transgender people change their sexuality when they transition.
* Gender is universal.
* All drag queens and kings are transgender.

* Surgery is a top priority for all transgender people, gender nonconforming.
* Insurers don't have to cover transition-related care.

Although there has been a small shift in cultural acceptance of those who are trans or gender diverse, society as a whole is a long way from acceptance. At the very least, trans people want to be viewed as part of the natural spectrum of human diversity. Unfortunately, because the concept of a trans person is confusing, at best, to most "straight" people, women and men—*young* women and men, especially—are confused as to whom to reach out to regarding issues of gender dysphoria.

Primary health care professionals have to be comfortable in caring for these patients and in dealing with the psychosocial complexities specific to their journeys. A clinician should be the quarterback in referring patients suffering from gender dysphoria to the right mental health care professionals—namely, doctors that specialize in gender-affirming counseling and/or hormonal therapy.

As of late, research shows that 24 percent of transgender persons report unequal treatment in health care environments and 19 percent report refusal of care altogether. Not surprisingly, a third of transgender persons do not seek preventative care at all. Health care needs of the transgender community are simply not given the attention they deserve.

I met Ryan, a handsome, slight-built twenty-eight-year-old man—who reminded me of a young Johnny Depp—at the behest of his mother, whom I'd known for twenty years. She'd called to ask if I would be comfortable seeing her transgender son, since he'd recently had horrible visits with a very insensitive gynecologist. Ryan had a long history of debilitating menstrual cramps, such that he wanted a hysterectomy to end his misery. He also told me that he and his mother had been very close.

Ryan:

> *"My father was abusive. My mom and I forged a strong relationship as we banded together in the face of this trauma. I came out to her as trans last year, about a month before she was due to come out to L.A. to visit me. She seemed to take it well enough, but a few days later, my younger sibling informed me that my mother had said what I was doing was evil. She also said that being an unattractive female was not reason enough to transition to male! Clearly, she didn't understand. I talked to her about how hurt I was by her comments. Our relationship has slowly been getting better. I'm told she now sometimes uses my real name (not my given name) when she refers to me. But she has asked me not to obtain medical care with permanent effects. Of course, I support myself and I'm old enough to do as I wish, which I will.*
>
> *Sometimes I'm sad I didn't transition when I was younger, for the sake of my physical self, but, when I consider the emotional damage my mother's resistance and horror may have caused me at a younger age, it makes me glad that I came to my realizations about transitioning later in life, when I had control over my medical options."*

## Family Acceptance or Lack Thereof

Transgender: It's not a phase, it's not a disease; it's a variance.

As with Ryan's mother, parents often struggle with dealing with a young son who prefers a pink tutu to a cowboy outfit, or dressing up as Jasmine over Aladdin. They may worry when a daughter chooses a Teenage Mutant Ninja Turtles-themed birthday party instead of one awash in pinks and ballerinas.

Family dynamics are complicated, even for those who are not transgender. Family *beliefs* are deeply rooted in tradition, religion, and culture. According to the Family Acceptance Project (FAP), "Many families believe they are helping their children by discouraging them from being true to who they know themselves to be, whether in relation to their gender identity or gender expression." FAP found, "When families did not feel judged for their religion or their beliefs, but were met where they were, parents and other caregivers were more likely to move towards accepting their children's identity. Their approach assumes that families love their children and want them to have a good life."

It has been noted that families that accept their transgender youth have less mental health and substance abuse issues and less suicide attempts among their children. In fact, FAP discovered that LGBTQ youth whose families affirm their gender identity and sexual orientation are almost *50 percent* less likely to attempt suicide than those youth of unsupportive families. It is now documented that family acceptance saves lives.

Although difficult, it is supremely important for parents and families to support their children's individualities and teach them to embrace their differences.

The transgender persons I spoke with for this section certainly back me up.

Will, a trans man:

> *"What a difference it can make having a supportive family. In fact, I have been extremely lucky to have a loving and accepting family and circle of friends, as well as a loving partner. My parents have always been open-minded and not defined by traditional gender roles, so it was easy for them to accept my transition.*
>
> *I often get the well-meaning, though misguided compliment that I look so good or that people 'can't even tell I'm trans.' When trans people are told this, what we often hear is 'you look good because you look like a cis person' or 'trans people who don't fit into cis-hetero expectations of beauty are ugly.' This puts the trans person in the awkward position of having to simultaneously thank and educate, or to throw the rest of the community under the bus if they don't explain why this kind of thinking can be hurtful."*

## Puberty Concerns

T.C. is a nineteen-year-old trans man whom I delivered. He talked to me about puberty, his first as a girl—with the hormones he was born with—and his "2nd puberty" when he was beginning hormones.

> *"I hated dresses from a young age. As I got curves, I felt more and more distant from my body. I wore collared shirts and pants to try and hide those curves. I slouched so as not to call attention to my chest. I don't even think I was really aware of my worsening posture. But, because I didn't know who I was at the time, my puberty felt like a normal rite of passage—nothing strange or dysphoria inducing."*

Out as trans, but not through 2nd puberty:

*"My periods became emotionally detrimental. I felt like my body was at war with my mind. Every time I menstruated, it was a reminder that I was born in the wrong body. I felt detached from myself. Getting out of the shower and seeing my reflection in the mirror was also difficult. I'd be reminded of all of the things that were wrong with my body."*

2nd puberty during hormone injections:

*"The hardest things about a second puberty were that I was breaking out everywhere, I was constantly irritable, hungry, and horny, I was having hot flashes, migraines, and irregular sleep because my body was actually being thrust into menopause. I am proud of myself for dealing with it all while going through high school, since that is arguably the worst time in any kid's life, but there were a few road bumps along the way. Because I was surer of my identity than most of my peers, I often felt disconnected from them. Whereas I was socially advanced, they were stunted. I felt trapped in a gray zone. The guys didn't see me as one of them and the girls didn't see me as a potential romantic partner. The more I worked out, the more prominent my facial hair and the lower my voice became, the more confident I felt...I still have some anxiety, but I am stronger for the experience."*

Transgender actor and filmmaker Jake Graf created a five-minute documentary called *Listen,* featuring young trans actors discussing the challenges they face at home, school, and in their personal lives. This documentary is a must-see if you want to experience what a group of eleven-to-fifteen-year-olds feel about growing up trans and the conflicts they face.

One story features a young girl having to listen to her parents fighting about who caused her gender identity problems, while another boy won't eat or drink, so he won't need to go to the bathroom, where he'll certainly face teasing or worse. Another teen cries in front of their mirror in fear of how puberty will affect their body if they aren't allowed hormone blockers.

Graf is a leader in helping to increase the visibility of trans children and allowing their voices to be heard. He has said, "Trans children are attacked so frequently that most feel powerless to stand up and be heard. We hope this film gives a voice to all transgender children and begins the much needed conversations about positive progress."

Anonymous trans woman:

*"When I was four, I noticed my sisters being called pretty, while I was called handsome, and it broke my heart. When I was about twelve, I found the words for how I felt and that's when I knew I was really a girl. By fourteen, I made sure all my friends knew it as well. At seventeen, I came out to my mother as a woman and a lesbian, and I started medically transitioning. I was fortunate enough to get the chance to start my second puberty before the first was completed. Where I wasn't so lucky was in having to go through my transition in the environment of a conservative Christian school with strict rules regarding gender presentation.*

*Throughout middle and high school, it was clear my body was betraying me. I fought it every way I could. I'd have friends put makeup on me at Sephora. I shaved my entire body from the cheekbones down and regularly had my eyebrows done. I found most of my solace in goth/ punk subcultures and anime, where boys were allowed to be pretty and feminine. Suffice to say, my preferences didn't make me popular in an evangelical environment, but I didn't care because I felt closer to being the girl I knew I was.*

*I transitioned just before positive trans representation began to proliferate in mainstream media, which means I grew up searching for any story or reference in pop culture that featured the life I wanted to lead. Unfortunately, everything I found terrified me. Almost every movie or TV show featuring trans women treated those women as less than people—as freaks or confused gay men, tragic people to be laughed at or killed. Before reaching adulthood, I was told that happiness, success, and romantic love would be inaccessible to me as a trans person. If it weren't for sites like tumblr and YouTube, which trans women use as platforms to share their own experiences, I would have been too scared to transition.*

*It has been eight years since I transitioned. I've spent those years building a career as a creative person that educates others on queer sexuality and dating. In my professional life, very few people know that I'm transgender, but, in my private life, I've been blessed to have fellow queer and gay women, both cis and trans, as community, friends, family, lovers, and partners who accept me for all of who I am. I still have insecurities about my womanhood, my body, and how the world sees me, but I've come to realize that those insecurities are common not just for trans women, but all women."*

Puberty can be a pivotal and traumatic time in the life of a trans woman or man. Biologically pre-programmed hormonal changes in puberty are usually in opposition to the identity of a trans person. Estrogen and testosterone flood the body on autopilot, giving development to a vagina or penis, along with pubic hair (and chest and facial hair for males). Often, trans girls and boys want hormones for puberty suppression—which is exactly what it sounds like, hormonal treatment for preventing development of secondary sex characteristics. It's felt that hormonal affirming care should *not* be delayed until gender stability is established. Ideally, hormone-blocking medication would be available to these trans children in order to stop puberty, thus preventing them from being further traumatized by the hormonal effects of the wrong gender identity.

Will:

> *"When I started going through puberty, I didn't even know that transgender people existed. I didn't think it particularly strange that I didn't want to have a menstrual cycle. In 2012, I started taking hormones about a year after I came out as a transgender man. The effects were exciting because I started seeing myself as I'd always imagined myself looking. I felt validated, and relieved of my dysphoria. This year, I'll have been on testosterone for seven years, and I don't believe I've had any negative side effects. The one challenge I had was as a singer in my college's chorus. I was learning Beethoven's 9th Symphony with a vocal range that was rapidly dropping lower and temporarily shrinking. Just like a cisgender boy going through puberty, my voice would crack. At one point, the whole top part of my vocal range disappeared. It eventually came back, and I developed a falsetto. Fortunately, that was the worst that happened as a result of the testosterone. But I do know that each gender journey is unique!"*

## Medical Transition

For trans women, hormone replacement therapy can be as necessary a part of the medical transition as testosterone is for trans men, in which case, an endocrinologist who specializes in trans care is the expert needed to guide trans women and men through the transition process sensitively and safely.

Beyond hormone therapy is surgery, which is often necessary in treating gender dysphoria. Left untreated, gender dysphoria can cause depression, anxiety, self-injury, and suicide—in that sense, treatment is often a matter of life and death. The overall goal of treatment is to fix the psychological and emotional distress associated with dysphoria. Insurance companies do, in fact, cover many aspects of medical treatments as well as provide coverage for transition-related care. In fact, insurance companies cannot deny transition care, because it is illegal to do so.

### *Gender Affirmation Surgery (GAS)*

What's important to understand is that having a vagina or penis no longer defines gender identity. Having top or bottom surgery is not always a priority. Not every trans women or man can afford surgery or even wants to have surgery. Aside from that, there is no one "right way" to do a medical or surgical transition. Sex reassignment surgery is a very expensive proposition, and the truth is that trans people, as a group, are known to have high unemployment rates, which makes it particularly difficult for many to surgically transition.

Certain states, such as California and New York, require insurers to cover transgender care. Countries like Canada and the United Kingdom will cover bottom surgery under nationalized health care.

### *Top Surgery*

Trans men usually want to do a bilateral mastectomy to remove the breast tissue, and then have chest contouring to help make the chest more male-shaped. Reconstructing the nipples and areolas is often part of top surgery.

For trans women, an appearance of a female chest can occur by placing breast implants underneath the natural breast tissue and muscle. Some trans women often benefit by having fat transferred from the belly, hips, or thighs to help make the breast area appear more full.

### *Bottom Surgery...What Does That Actually Mean?*

Transfeminine bottom surgery refers to one of the many surgical techniques in the transformation of male genitalia as it is reconstructed into that of a female.

Vaginoplasty refers to the surgery typically pursued by transgender women and AMAB (assigned male at birth) non-binary people. Specifically, there are three main ways to create a vagina, including penile inversion, rectosigmoid or colon graft, and non-penile inversion vaginoplasty. In all three of these types of vaginoplasty, the clitoris is created from the head of the penis.

Interestingly enough, some trans women do not find that a vagina necessarily "makes the woman." In fact, Sasha Clary, a trans woman wrote a fascinating article called "Having a Vagina Really Mattered...Until I Got One." In the article, Sasha explains:

*"In a way, having a vagina means nothing to me. It's the relief from body dysmorphia that makes all the difference, the freedom from having a body configured in such a way that doesn't make sense to me. Do I feel more 'complete' now? I suppose I could say that. But having a vagina is only one small part of it. Transgender life experience encompasses so much more than any one body part could ever summarize. I felt conviction that I was female when I was very young. I felt that same conviction when I was an adult, before medical intervention. I feel that same conviction now, and surgery had no effect on it. Not all transgender people feel this same arc. No two transgender people conceive of themselves in the same way. But my perception of myself isn't uncommon. More than anything, social and medical transition have made it so the outside world understands me better, rather than conforming or changing myself into something different than I was.... Society has an unhealthy obsession with genitals and body parts."*

Sasha goes on to say that she ended up having vaginoplasty *"for simple convenience. I wanted to be free from the inconvenience of tucking and strapping down my previous body parts to keep them out of sight. I wanted to feel pretty in a bathing suit."*

Lindsey D. also shared her experiences with GAS:

*"'Did it turn out OK? Does everything look OK?' I believe those were the first words I said upon waking up after revision surgery—six months ago after my original vaginoplasty...[But] my neo trans vagina is a masterpiece of art. Not sculpted by the hand of God, but by the hands of two Wonder Woman bandana-wearing Goddesses!*

*The best surgeons! Two female surgeons. Two amazing doctors with the utmost concern for my health, my well-being, and my happiness. They performed a clitoralplasty, labiaplasty, and an urethroplasty that took about an hour and half in the operating room.*

*For many years, it has been taboo within and without the trans community to talk about our genitalia because of all of the violence and politics that go with it. We trans folk have long resisted answering any questions about our anatomy responding with, 'It's none of your business. I would never ask you about what's going on between your legs.' But the truth is, it is what's going on between our legs that's getting us trans people killed. Especially trans women of color. The sooner that everyone, most of all, men, understand that it doesn't matter at ALL what's between our legs, that we pee and poop like everybody else; the sooner we might stem much of the anti-trans violence."*

## For Trans Men

Phalloplasty and metoidioplasty are two procedures typically pursued by transgender men and AFAM (assigned female at birth) nonbinary people.

During a metoidioplasty the clitoral hood is removed to allow the clitoris to grow and act as a small penis. Other surgical changes may include lengthening the urethral so that the patient can urinate out of the newly formed penis. The vaginal opening can then be closed, and prosthetic testicles can be placed to create male genitalia.

During a phalloplasty a penis is created using skin from another part of the body.

Brody's journey describes the commitment in this particular transformation.

Brody L. Fitzpatrick, trans male:

*"I had the first stage of Radial Forearm Flap Phalloplasty with Dr. Maurice Garcia of Cedar Sinai Hospital in Los Angeles on January 29, 2018, stage two June 6, 2018 and stage three on March 27, 2019.*

*"I began to prepare for the physical changes and emotional/spiritual challenges months in advance. I felt anxious and worried about infections and complications. My biggest fears were how it would affect me sexually and whether anyone would want to be intimate with me after the surgery. I felt guilt and privilege that my insurance covered it. I spent time validating, affirming, and forgiving. I prayed, maintained a healthy diet and continued to work out. Two weeks before surgery, I began to have nightmares that my penis was grabbed and torn from my body.*

*"On the day of surgery, I was relaxed and placed my trust in the hands of Dr. Garcia and his surgical team. Everything went well, with no complications, and I began to prepare for stage two. I couldn't wait to move forward because it was becoming increasingly uncomfortable having both a penis and vagina. The stakes were significantly higher with the second stage, but I felt confident in my daily practice and continued to trust. Fortunately, everything healed well and there were no serious complications. I am able to feel aroused, can orgasm, and, more importantly, had a successful sexual encounter.*

> *"I intentionally waited eight months before the third stage because I needed a break from surgery to spend time 'doing me.' I am presently recovering from getting testicular prosthetics. A cis male apologized for not telling me before surgery that testicles are uncomfortable. It's a welcome discomfort to have, as far as I'm concerned, and I'm proud of my complete package.*
>
> *"I am excited to move forward with the final stage, which will enable me to have intercourse. I feel extremely fortunate to have had this life-altering, saving, and enhancing experience."*

As you can see, there were many stages in Brody's journey to becoming male. In order to make it clearer to the trans "lay-person," so to speak, his journey is broken down here:

## *Stage 1*

* A full thickness graft is harvested—meaning complete epidermis and dermis—from the patient, one from the back of each thigh (where leg meets buttocks).
* A flap of skin is harvested from a forearm and used to create a urethra and phallus.
* Phallus is then attached to the body, connecting the blood vessels and a harvested nerve.

**Total surgery time:** 13 hours

**Hospital stay:** Nine to ten days. However, the graft takes about a year before it is completely healed.

### *Stage 2*

* Complete Hysterectomy.
* Vaginectomy, the surgical removal of all or part of the vagina.
* Scrotoplasty, one of several operations performed to transform/reform the external genitalia into a penis and a scrotum.
* Urethra hook-up.
* Glansplasty, the procedure that creates a glans and coronal ridge on the penis.
* Clitoral Transposition – meaning that the clitoris is transposed, buried, and fixed directly below the reconstructed phallic shaft.

**Total surgery time:** Eleven hours

**Hospital stay:** Four days, followed by six to eight weeks of limited activity

### *Stage 3*

* Testicular implants in scrotum

**Total surgery time:** Ninety minutes

**Hospital stay:** Overnight, and limited activities for six weeks

### *Stage 4*

* Pump for erectile dysfunction

**Hospital stay:** Four to five days with limited activity for up to eight weeks

From Will, a trans man:

*"I am not considering bottom surgery, with the exception of a hysterectomy. The majority of the dysphoria I experienced was tied to my chest, and having people gender me in a way that didn't align with how I know myself to be. While there are some things related to my genitals that will bother me every once in a while, the options for bottom surgeries aren't worth the cost or healing process for me. There are some sex-related bottom dysphoria issues I have, but nothing worth paying thousands of dollars for. I do want to get a hysterectomy eventually, not for any validation of my manhood, but due to the fear that testosterone could become unavailable or harder to get some day—in which case, I would have estrogen take over as my main sex hormone and begin having a menstrual cycle again."*

For many trans women and men, bottom surgery is not the be all and end all, but, for those who want their genitals to reflect their sexual identity as male or female, it is a viable option—if one can afford it.

In the case of bottom surgery, a big question is whether or not one can experience an orgasm after such a surgery. A study done in Karolinska University in Sweden found that up to five years post-surgery, the vast majority of trans women were orgasmic, as well as generally satisfied with their surgery. Any post-surgical numbness improved with time, and orgasms could be achieved through direct clitoral stimulation and or vaginal penetration.

For trans men opting for a metoidioplasty—a procedure that removes the clitoral hood in order to allow the clitoris to be a small penis—sexual function is typically not affected since there are no nerves cut during metoidioplasty. Additionally, trans men take testosterone, which makes the clitoris grow from one to three inches.

Unfortunately, despite all the advances in surgical techniques and procedures, the one thing surgery cannot help are the feelings of anxiety and depression that many trans people face, especially trans youth.

## Mental Illness—An Unfair Deck

Leelah Alcorn was a seventeen-year-old trans woman who took her life because she felt unaccepted by her parents. She felt there was no way out of her anxiety and depression. Before she died, she wrote: "The life I would've lived isn't worth living in...because I'm transgender...."

The suicide rate in the trans community is *41 percent.* It is no secret, as well, that transgender youth are at a much higher risk of mental illness—including depression, anxiety, self-harm, and suicidal thoughts—than the cis population. A recent 2015 study led by Sari L. Reisner from the Harvard T. H. Chan School of Public Health determined the need for "gender-affirming mental health services and intervention to support transgender youth."

Because pediatricians are the first health care providers transgender children are exposed to, they must be on the front line of those sensitive, gender-affirming services. Reisner's study states: "If transgender children cannot be seen for who they are it can be very distressing."

If you or someone you know is in emotional crisis or at risk of suicide, there are places and people that can help.

* The National Suicide Prevention Lifeline: 1-800-273-8255.
* The Trevor Project: a twenty-four-hour crisis hotline that provides support for LGBTQ youth: 1-866-488-7386.
* The Trans Lifeline: (877) 565-8860

## Conversion Therapy...Does NOT Work!

Conversion therapy, also referred to as "reparative therapy," involves dangerous nontraditional practices that "falsely claim to change a person's sexual orientation or gender identity or expression" according to the Human Rights Campaign (HRC). The HRC condemns such therapy, and goes on to say, "Such practices have been rejected by every mainstream medical and mental health organization for decades, but due to continuing discrimination and societal bias against LGBTQ people, some practitioners continue to conduct conversion therapy."

Fortunately, laws are being discussed to outlaw conversation therapy, and many states, including California, Connecticut, Nevada, New Jersey, the District of Columbia, Oregon, Illinois, Vermont, New York, New Mexico, Rhode Island, Washington, Hawaii, Maryland, New Hampshire, and Delaware, have already set an example by creating regulations protecting LGBTQ youth from this dangerous, barbaric, and antiquated practice. Those states are encouraging schools to teach students at an early age what transgender means.

Schools must be at the forefront of educating children and teaching tolerance. Transgender youth must know that it is okay for them to be the way they are. HRC goes on to remind us that Psychiatrist Dr. L. Spitzer, a noted psychiatry giant who once offered a study on reparative therapy, recanted his findings late in his life and apologized for endorsing the practice.

Trans men and women want to get the message out that they are no different in their physical and emotional needs and in their humanity than the rest of the population. If anything, they are more in tune to emotional and psychological suffering.

Will has said to me:

> *"If I could tell my younger self something, it would be to not try to change myself for anyone else's benefit. Anyone who doesn't love you for who you are isn't worth your time.*
>
> *It's important for people to remember that there is no one way to be any gender, man, woman, or any sort of non-binary identity. Trans people don't all seek medical transition, and it doesn't invalidate their experience or their identity. Sometimes people don't have the financial or logistical access to the medical procedures they'd like, and sometimes people don't feel like the changes that would come with those procedures are necessary to be their most authentic selves. Trans folks shouldn't be judged on how masculine, feminine, or cisgender-passing they are. We, just like anyone else, want to be able to live a safe and healthy life."*

Society is slowly trying to understand the complexities and nuances of the trans community, but acceptance by the majority is difficult. As a health care provider, I want to help others understand the many medical and social realities of this marginalized group of people. With knowledge and education come truth, compassion, and wisdom and an unraveling of the cultural bias, discrimination, and myths surrounding *all* marginalized people. Bias is oftentimes unconscious, and stereotypes abound. We've all seen how easy it is for certain media outlets and political circles to perpetuate myth and spread wrong information (if not lies).

Simply, as with any group of people, respect and dignity is the goal of the trans community. And, of course, acceptance.

I like to believe and support the idea that knowledge leads to wisdom and tolerance. Respect and dignity are the goals of trans persons. Education is knowledge. And, after all, love is love.

In the words of Leelah Alcorn, the seventeen-year-old trans woman who took her own life: "My death has to mean something; my death needs to be counted. Fix society please."

I believe we can do this. All of us together.

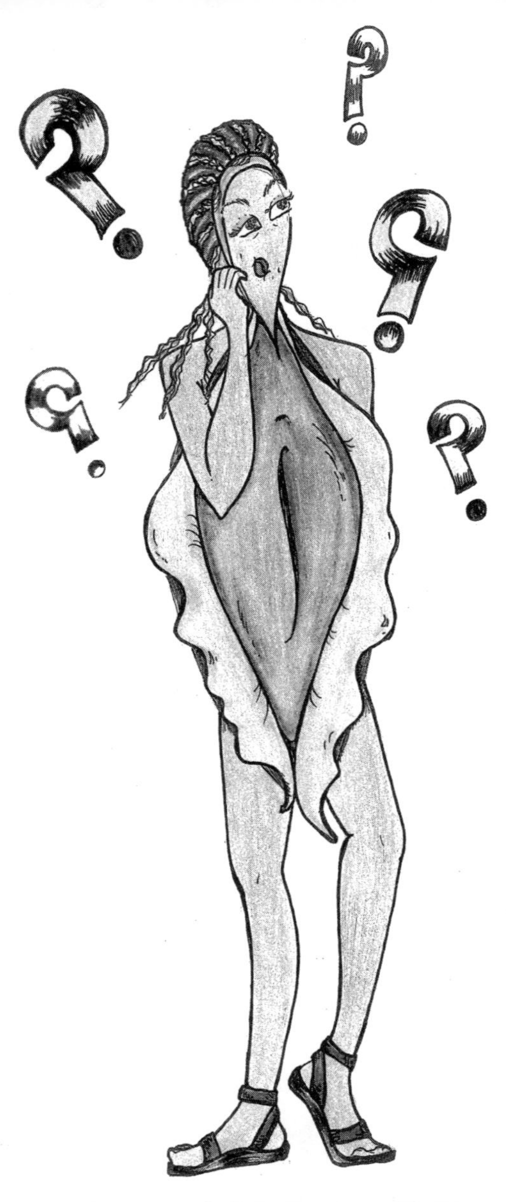

CHAPTER 15

# confused

"Dr. Sherry is the best. Few people have as much experience and expertise as she has. I have been so lucky to be her patient and to have had access to her seemingly endless knowledge. Now readers can have access to that knowledge as well, because she also happens to be a great writer."

—**Zooey Deschanel** Actress and Singer-Songwriter

Health myths. They're still out there, and still run rampant. Case in point: How many times have you looked to "Dr. Google" or a relative or best friend for medical advice? Be honest now, because you're not alone! So many women wind up getting their medical information from sources outside their doctor's office, which is one of the best ways to create confusion around a topic or—worst-case scenario—venture into dangerous medical complications.

I know, I know, with so much vagina information on the internet and so many things to do in a day, it seems like a no-brainer to save time searching via Google for the ten top diagnoses of, say, vaginal itch. And, certainly, even though #10 is vulvar cancer, you go straight to that diagnosis and convince yourself that you need complete removal of your outer vagina in order to treat the itch. Believe me, this is not a stretch. I've had patients come into my office after a self-diagnosis of cancer, when, actually, what they are dealing with is a run-of-the-mill yeast infection or irritation from a new soap.

Let's face it: Vaginas are complicated. To many—men and women alike—they are often a complete mystery, which is why I want to explore the most common questions and myths I hear when a patient is in my examination room with her feet up in the stirrups. I've divided this chapter into three sections in order to break down the different categories of questioning. To that end, first up is:

## Confusion About the Vagina's Care and Maintenance

### *V-A-G-I-N-A. What's in a Name?*

Sure, you say, I know what it's called, and I know how to spell it, but the truth is that most women do not refer to their vaginas with the word "vagina." I've heard it referred to—even in my office—as everything from "south of the belly button" to "down there" to "va-jay-jay" and "cooch." As much as I'd love for the word "vagina" to roll trippingly off a woman's tongue, I understand that most women are more comfortable using nicknames. However, when it comes to hygiene and health, it's important to understand and be able to correctly identify all the different *parts* of the vagina.

Your vagina is actually the muscular canal that connects the cervix and uterus to the outside world. And talk about flexibility, that particular muscle can stretch large enough to allow a baby through it. Hello, world!

The outside of the vagina is referred to as the vulva, and includes the lips or labia minora (small lips), labia majora (larger lips), introitus (the opening of the vagina), the clitoris, and the urethra (where urine comes out). These terms are important to know so that you can be specific in referring to any problems "down there."

When patients come to me with concerns such as itching, swelling, and pimples of the vagina, the problem is usually with the vulva or labia. So it's important to know what your "best girlfriend" (yes, that's another term I've heard for vagina) actually looks like in order to be able to talk clearly about *her* different parts. My advice always is to grab a mirror and take a good look "under the hood!" Go ahead and identify all those parts for yourself.

### *To Clean or Not to Clean, That Is the Question*

You may have heard the old adage that the vagina is "self-cleaning," but your vagina needs the same hygienic attention you would give to your face or, for that matter, any other part of your body. Between the residue of urine and sweat and the vagina's close proximity to the anus, it is critical to keep clean the outside of the vagina (the labia minora and majora) in order to prevent the kind of bacterial buildup that may lead to pimples, acne, offensive odors, and itching. The vagina's sweat glands and hair follicles are just as prone to dirt buildup as any other part of the body.

If you give the same care and attention to your vagina as you would to your face—such as properly cleansing, hydrating, and moisturizing—the ultra-sensitive and delicate skin of your vagina will age in a much healthier way.

So, yes, the answer to the question is, inarguably, *to clean*. That said, the best method is to use non-fragrant soap and water on the labia every day. You may use two fingers to gently clean the vaginal opening, and then go one to two knuckles into the opening with the same gentle, non-fragranced soap.

Along those lines, it is important to know what kind of cleaning you *don't* need. I'm talking about douching. Hard to believe, but one in four women still douche regularly—maybe it's a holdout from all those '70s commercials encouraging "feminine hygiene"—but the truth is that douching is not only unnecessary it can increase your risk of yeast and bacterial infections. Douches and scented feminine cleansers actually do more harm than good by disrupting the natural balance of the healthy bacteria that prevent infections. Stay away from them, even if your mother or grandmother swears by them.

### *Dehydration Down There*

Dry skin is uncomfortable and annoying on any part of one's body, but it is especially so when it comes to the sensitive skin of the vagina. The vagina and labia are as susceptible to dryness as the skin on any other part of your body. As your skin and overall health benefit when your body is properly hydrated, the skin of the vagina benefits as well. Proper hydration helps to keep the labia moist and lubricated, as prevention against the pain and itching of dry skin.

On the subject of proper hydration, I like to remind my patients that water is vital for every system in our body—it makes up 60 percent of our body weight—so constant replenishment is *essential*. I'm often asked what *amount* of water is necessary to consume each day. The answer depends upon how active you are, your medical history, and the climate in which you live. In general, though, you need to drink at least eight 8-ounce glasses—or two liters—of water daily and consume alcohol and caffeine in moderation, as both those substances tend to be big moisture suckers.

A handful of extra virgin coconut oil tossed into a warm bath, three to four times a week, is a great way to rehydrate the skin of the vagina—and it's not so bad for the rest of your body as well. The addition of oral or vaginal probiotics to your daily regimen can also serve to keep the vagina healthy, happy, and in harmony with the rest of your body.

## *Vaginal Discharge…What's Normal and What's Not?*

The vagina is equipped with over thirty organisms that help keep its natural pH balance, which aids in keeping it free of infection. These organisms produce *secretions*—in the form of vaginal discharge—much like the mouth does with saliva and the eyes do with tears. (Maybe we should think of that discharge as saliva for the vagina! Just a thought.) The cervical glands also contribute to the vaginal secretions, and, depending on the time of the month, vaginal discharge may change in consistency, texture, and smell.

A couple days after the end of your period, your discharge will appear thick and white. Around Day Fourteen, you may notice a clear, slippery, odorless discharge, the consistency of egg whites. This is completely normal and suggests ovulation, the time when a woman may become pregnant.

During puberty, a milky, thin, odorless discharge (leukorrhea) is normally produced. This naturally occurring discharge protects the stability of the vagina and becomes thicker right before your period.

Throughout your cycle, if you should notice a strange new odor or vulvar itching, redness, burning or swelling, or an unusual change in color of your discharge, you may have cause for concern. A strong, foul, fishy vaginal odor accompanied by a thin, grayish-white discharge is a classic symptom of bacterial infection. It can also be a result of other types of organisms (infections) such as candidiasis (yeast infection), bacterial vaginosis/gardnerella (referring to an overgrowth of bacteria), Trichomoniasis or chlamydia (both common sexually transmitted diseases, or STDs), or even gonorrhea (a common STD that may often show no signs or symptoms).

Women often make the mistake of assuming that, if they're experiencing vaginal itching and discharge, it must be a yeast infection. Off to the drug store they go in order to buy an over-the-counter medication. Unfortunately, this can make the symptoms worse and delay proper diagnosis and treatment. It's only with a vaginal culture that you can receive confirmation of what type of organism (or infection) is causing your disruptive symptoms. And it's only with that proper identification that the best treatment may be prescribed.

When in doubt—and before you start putting yogurt into your vagina or attempting other hand-me-down remedies—be sure to see your health care provider in order to determine the exact nature of your vaginal pain or discomfort!

## *Period Odor*

Patients have told me: *I know I smell differently during my period. And I think my friends can smell it too!*

Yes, it's true that there may be a special "period odor" to your period but be assured that others can't smell it. Menstrual blood does have a unique smell, but the scent doesn't travel beyond your own "personal space." The scent is usually mild and should not be offensive or fishy-smelling. If, indeed, period blood comes in contact with unwanted bacteria in the vagina, and you notice a foul odor, chances are that an infection may be brewing. In such a case, best to see your health care provider.

## *Vaginal Sounds or Does a Vagina Fart?*

Yes, it does! And I'm here to tell you that vaginal "farts" are normal.

Many of us have—for lack of a better word—*noisy* vaginas. Whether you call that female phenomenon a fart, flatulence, fanny fart, vart, or queef, you are describing the particular sound that is made when air is released out of the vagina.

But how does air get into the vagina in the first place? Oftentimes it happens when fingers or a penis or sex toy go in and out of the vagina, bringing along additional air. Sex—specifically involving a penis—usually requires a lot of thrusting of the penis in and out of the vagina, which typically pushes extra air into that particular space. Not surprisingly, the only way for the air to escape is through the same door it came in, creating a sound that is not unlike the sound of gas being expelled from the rectum. There you have your vaginal *fart*.

Certain sex positions, such as doggy style and inverted missionary position, seem to increase the *queefing* effect. Therefore, it stands to reason that the best way to prevent queefing is to avoid putting anything in the vagina—which may or may not sound like a bit of a buzz kill. There are, however, other causes of queefing, which may include certain forms of exercise routines including yoga and stretching—again, avoiding those exercise routines may not be what you had in mind. Inserting tampons, diaphragms, and menstrual cups can all lead to a noisy vagina.

My advice is to try to laugh about those annoying queefs, because chances are that you are having fun creating those special vaginal sound effects.

### *Waxing vs. Shaving*

I tend to go with waxing as a means of getting rid of unwanted pubic hair. Waxing can have a kinder and gentler effect than shaving on the skin in the pubic area and can be safely done every four to six weeks. The trick is to make sure that the skin in this sensitive area is clean prior to any hair removal. Afterward, some gentle loofah action, combined with an antibacterial soap or lotion, can help prevent acne and ingrown hairs during the regrowth process.

### *On Achieving the Perfect Vagina*

First off, there is no such thing as the "perfect" vagina!

Unfortunately, our current cultural obsession with the perfect or ideal vagina is causing a lot of unfounded promises having to do with vaginal "rejuvenation." There are surgeries "guaranteed" to provide "revirgination" and "G-spot amplification," but vagina owners beware! The pursuit of a "designer vagina" is bound to result in less than satisfying, if not downright dangerous, results.

While some doctors do promote and recommend such surgical procedures, those procedures remain very controversial and are *not* supported by the American College of Obstetrics and Gynecology. In fact, they can result in permanent complications—including scarring, infection, and chronic pain. Always, *always,* get a second or third opinion from a reputable gynecologist before considering a procedure that you may someday regret.

## Confusion About Sex and the Vagina

### *What is Safe Sex?*

So let's say your partner *tells* you that they test "negative" for sexually transmitted infections, and, because of that, you don't need to use a condom. You take them at their word and have unprotected sex, right?

Wrong.

Safe sex—a term you've probably heard since you were old enough to *have* sex—means protecting yourself not only from unwanted pregnancy, but from STIs (sexually transmitted infections), also known as STDs (sexually transmitted diseases), and especially HPV (some types of which can lead to cancer).

According to the data released in the CDC's (Centers for Disease Control and Prevention) annual "Sexually Transmitted Disease Surveillance Report," the number of cases of chlamydia, gonorrhea, and syphilis in 2016 was the highest number recorded in this country's public health history. The more than two million reported cases set an alarming new record, with chlamydia leading the charge at approximately 1.6 million diagnoses.

For women especially, untreated STIs can lead to shattering, long-term complications such as infertility, stillbirth, and greater vulnerability to HIV infection. Rounding out the remainder of those STIs reported for 2016 includes HPV, herpes, HIV, trichomoniasis, hepatitis, and Zika virus. HPV, the most common of the STIs, affected 90 percent of women and 80 percent of men *once they became sexually active*.

Even if your partner goes to their doctor for an STI check-up and receives a clean bill of health, there is still a chance that you may contract an STI from them. Part of the reason for that is HPV and HSV are difficult to find during a routine checkup unless there is an active wart or lesion on the man's penis or the woman's vagina. A partner can transmit both these viruses through sexual contact, even if that partner tested "negative" during a physical exam.

Although regular condom use cannot *guarantee* 100 percent protection against sexually transmitted infections, it is still the best "safe sex" practice aside from abstinence.

## *Allergies to Condoms and Semen—Yes, it's Possible*

Okay, so one more time (because I can't stress this enough): A strict adherence to condom use is your best defense against unwanted STIs.

That said, a small percentage of women have latex allergies. And, since the majority of condoms today are made out of latex, that can result in vaginal swelling, itching, and pain for those women. If you find that you are in that small percentage, you may substitute a polyurethane condom. As in food, check the labels!

## Confused V

You can't check the "label" on semen, but, unfortunately, 20,000 to 40,000 women in the United States can be allergic to their partner's semen. Many specialists believe it's more common than reported, mainly because it is often undiagnosed or misdiagnosed. A semen allergy occurs when a woman produces antibodies against certain proteins found in the seminal fluid in a man's *ejaculate* (the fancy term for semen).

Symptoms are similar to those of STIs and may include redness, swelling, pain, itching, blisters, and/or a burning sensation in the vagina, often occurring 10–30 minutes after contact with the semen. Similar symptoms may appear in the mouth or on any other areas of the skin in touch with the semen. In extreme cases, a sufferer's entire body may be afflicted with hives and swelling, to the extent of difficulty in breathing or anaphylactic shock (similar to an allergic reaction to bee stings or peanuts).

A process of elimination often determines diagnosis of a semen allergy, since the symptoms can mirror those of yeast or herpes infections or allergies to latex, spermicides, lubricants, or feminine hygiene products. If you suspect an allergy is present, it is advisable to see an allergist that has experience with this particular problem. Treatment often involves identifying which proteins in the semen are causing the allergic reaction, and then using a desensitization process to build up tolerance. This can be accomplished through allergy shots containing small doses of your partner's semen, or by intra-vaginal insertion of small amounts of that same semen.

If a sperm allergy is, indeed, present, you shouldn't experience any symptoms if you use condoms and avoid any other contact with the semen. But, if that's not quite an option, at least you know that there is a treatment!

## *The Pleasure Principle or What Exactly Is an Orgasm Anyway?*

*Orgasm.* We all know (or have at least heard) that it's pleasurable to have one and that it's even beneficial to our health, but what exactly is an orgasm?

Well, women achieve sexual pleasure primarily from stimulation of the clitoris—that highly sensitive part of a woman's vagina, composed of millions of nerve endings similar to that of the penis. When your clitoris is touched, licked, caressed, or rubbed (with varying degrees of pressure), you may become sexually aroused, which can ultimately lead to orgasm.

With sexual arousal, there is an increased blood flow to the genitals and a tensing of the muscles throughout the body, particularly in the genitals. Orgasm actually reverses this process and returns your body to its pre-arousal state through a series of rhythmic contractions, which are felt in the vagina, uterus, anus, and pelvic floor.

It's up to you to determine what feels good and what degree of touch and exploration is most satisfying. It's up to you to find where, exactly, your G-spot is hiding. That elusive G-spot simply refers to the most erogenous zone of your vagina (more than likely, the clitoris), which, when stimulated, may lead to orgasm and female ejaculation.

With that in mind, masturbation is the perfect way for you to get in touch with your own sexual please, literally and figuratively.

### *Is it Normal Not to Orgasm During Sexual Intercourse?*

Whoever said that it is normal for a woman to orgasm during sexual intercourse, must have been...*a man.*

With its 8,000 highly sensitive nerve endings, the main function of the clitoris is to give pleasure. When stimulated, it becomes three times its size, bringing you to orgasm. A recent study found that only 18 percent of women are able to have an orgasm with vaginal penetration alone! The majority of women have a clitoral orgasm only during oral and manual stimulation of the clitoris, although, it is possible to have an orgasm through vaginal penetration alone.

Go ahead, experiment and see what works best for you! Practice makes orgasm.

### *Is Bigger Better?*

Most sexually experienced women are the first to say that bigger is not better when it comes to penis size and girth. Between the effects of vaginal tears and uncomfortable sexual positions, a big penis does not necessarily register high on the scale of sexual pleasure.

Although no man likes to think that his penis is *typical,* the typical penis size is 5.7 inches in length and 4.8 inches in diameter (girth). In reality, when women are asked what is most important in a partner, penis size is low on the list of priorities. Traits like honesty, a sense of humor, and lovability rank much higher than penis size. However, when pressed to make a choice between length and thickness, overall, women prefer a thicker penis as opposed to a longer one.

So there's your answer: Size doesn't matter...but a bit of girth won't hurt.

## *Masturbation. Is it for Sex Fiends?*

No. No. No. Next!

Seriously, let me first say that masturbation is a completely normal, common, and completely *healthy* activity. Masturbation is simply an act during which you touch or self-stimulate your genitals in order to achieve sexual arousal and pleasure—and, with any luck, achieve orgasm.

A recent study revealed that 89 percent of women and 95 percent of men masturbate. In fact, masturbation tends to be the very first sexual experience to bring on an orgasm for both sexes! In fact, it's much easier to have an orgasm through masturbation than with intercourse. Unfortunately, masturbation is a topic that is strictly off limits in some circles—ethnic, religious, social, you name it. The word alone can bring about embarrassment, shame, and anxiety.

Masturbation—seriously, try saying it out loud. And, once and for all, please remember how natural and normal (and satisfying) it is.

## *The Ultimate Lube Job*

Why is it we know more about the importance of lubing our cars than we do about lubing our vaginas?

Vaginal lubrications are great accompaniments for most sexual activities for women of any age, *especially* if you experience vaginal dryness and/or discomfort with sex. Simply, lubes can make sex more fun!

The best lubrications are water-based and unscented, which are easier on the vagina and tend to cause less irritation than alcohol-based and heavily perfumed ones. K-Y Jelly—the original one and only—and still one of the best lubrications on the market, remains the most reliable and the least likely to cause irritation or allergic reaction.

Another lubrication option is extra virgin coconut oil, which is one of the most multi-functional oils around. It is not only good for hydrating skin, but it is a great lubricant for sex. Men love how it feels on the penis and women love how it feels in the vagina—it's a win-win for both genders.

As for other oil-based lubes, some can destroy latex condoms, so best to read the fine print on the wrapper (sounds like I'm talking about a candy, doesn't it?). Silicone-based lubes feel good and make for a satisfying amount of slipping and sliding, but they can break down silicone sex toys.

Depending on your preference (and your condom or toy), there are many lubricant choices available. Gotta love a lube.

### *If You Want to Watch Porn...That Is Your Prerogative*

BUT, don't mistake it for "normal" sexual activity or something you need aspire to!

With porn on the rise, our perception of what is "normal" sex is based on the skills and proclivities of Jenna Jameson, et al. No one seems to want to discuss how this new prevalence is resulting in misconceptions about sex or how it's changing our romantic and sexual relationships—not to mention our relationships to our own bodies.

Porn has taught an entire generation of women to hypersexualize and pornify themselves in their sexual relationships. It has created an epidemic of new, unattainable aesthetics. Do not let those aesthetics become your new normal of what ought to happen under the sheets.

Porn is sexual fantasy, not sexual reality. Important to know the difference!

### *When is it Too Late to "Change My Mind?"*

The short answer: Never. It is never too late to change your mind about engaging in sex. Period.

Sex must always be consensual. Again, if you are uncomfortable, it is never ever too late to say no to sexual activity with your partner. That much I hope we've all learned from these past couple years.

### *Isn't Anal Sex Dirty?*

That's a trick question, ladies.

Let me put it this way: Yes, anal sex can be good, "naughty" fun, but it takes a certain amount of cleanliness. No matter how clean you think your anal area is, fecal matter and E. Coli lurk in and around the surface.

The risk of Hepatitis A and B is the main concern if E. Coli is ingested orally. Other "bad" bacteria and parasites in and around the anus include salmonella and C. difficile (a bacterium that causes diarrhea), so, if your partner has an active infection by any one of those harmful "bugs," and they are ingested during analingus—or what is commonly referred to as rimming—you may experience diarrhea, stomach pains, or a host of other intestinal problems.

If you plan on having sexual contact in the anal area, whether it is via tongue, finger, sex toy, or penis, you need to use warm water and soap (or baby wipes) to clean the area thoroughly *before* engaging in any contact.

Despite what you may have heard, there is no need for an enema or full bowel prep before engaging in any anal activity. But, if you want to clean the lower rectum, you can use an over-the-counter enema bulb with warm water to rinse out that area. Some people like to use latex gloves when doing digital exploring, but a good hand washing is enough protection. Shaving or waxing the anus before sexual contact is always an option, but this is a personal choice and not a necessity from a medical standpoint.

As far as readying yourself for anal sex, being mentally prepared is half the battle. Because the anal opening is much smaller and tighter than the vaginal opening, many women find anal penetration—with fingers or a penis—painful, no matter how adequately lubricated. You may want to first explore the sensation of anal penetration with a finger—yours or your partner's—or by using a sex toy. This will help to stretch the anal opening. Once that happens, you may be able to move on to more fingers, a penis, or bigger toys!

If you are of the small percentage of women who prefer anal sex, just make sure you take the time to loosen the muscles around the anus and to use plenty of lubrication. And don't forget those condoms.

## *I Can't Get an STD in Anal Sex*

*&*#. That's the buzzer for "wrong answer."

Yes, you can contract any variety of STIs from anal sex. Unfortunately, because it's not possible to get pregnant through anal sex, men and women alike make the mistake of thinking that they are "protected" during anal sex. The only protection you may have is against pregnancy. Unprotected sex means unsafe sex.

Have your partner wear a condom no matter which "door" you're using. It's your responsibility to prevent the risk of herpes, HPV, syphilis, and HIV transmission. Take charge.

### *Sex Toys Are a Girl's Best Friend*

If you haven't already discovered the myriad of sex toys available to women, I say: Treat yourself to a stroll around an online women's sex toy shop and pick up a little something for yourself.

Toys can help promote blood flow to the clitoris (and its 8,000 nerve endings) and add to your sexual responses and enjoyment—with or without a partner. Indeed, for many women, sex toys are a "best friend." Every day, new and improved toys are created and marketed, but, because the sex toy store industry is unregulated by the government, it's a little bit like the Wild West out there, which is why it's important to make sure that the toys you buy are safe and free of toxic chemicals such as polyvinyl chloride (PVC) or phthalates. Also, you want to make sure that your sex toys are not causing trauma to any parts of your vagina (or anus). Always, always wash your toys with warm water and soap in between using. Lastly, sex toys, much like toothbrushes, are not meant to be shared!

My favorite tried-and-true online shop (and F.A.O. Schwartz of sex toys) is calexotics.com, and my favorite sexual health and wellness site is sexualwellness.com. Take a stroll through both of them. I promise you won't be disappointed. In fact, you will definitely gain important sexual wellness information for your effort.

### *Loss of Libido*

Libido: sexual desire; sex drive; sexual longing—in psychoanalysis, it's the energy of the sexual drive as a component of the life instinct. It's no wonder that losing it can be one of the most frustrating and complicated challenges a woman deals with in her lifetime.

As important as sexual health is, addressing it is quite often not at the top of most women's "to do" list. Between work, financial stress, relationship obstacles, and the always-fraught bedtime choice of sleep over sex, women can definitely feel as though they have lost their drive. In addition to that laundry list of culprits, try adding certain medication, such as the birth control pill and antidepressants, both of which can add to the urge for a Netflix marathon rather than any sort of sexual encounter.

Talking about all this—sex and sexual desire and a lack thereof—is usually not a comfortable conversation for a woman to have with her best friend or partner, let alone a health care provider, yet it is an important conversation to have! Would you believe that nearly 50 percent of women never even broach the subject with their doctors?

Don't let loss of libido become a "given" in your life. Find a health care provider to talk to about it. It's worth your effort... for your mental and physical health, and for your overall sense of self.

## Confusion About Birth Control

### *The Withdrawal Method*

You would not believe how many women believe this to be a reliable form of birth control. I know this, because I am an OB-GYN who has dealt with the results of such form of birth control. Can you say "pregnancy?"

Even if your best, smartest girlfriend tells you it is reliable, and even if your mother or grandmother tells you they swore by that method, please do not rely on it if you want to ensure yourself against pregnancy. After all, there's a reason why it's called "the pull and pray method!"

During sex, and right before ejaculation, your partner can release some fluid called "pre-ejaculation." That pre-ejaculatory fluid may actually contain some active and viable sperm—in short, the kind of sperm that can make you pregnant.

### *Period Pregnancy*

Were you under the impression that you couldn't get pregnant while on your period? Well, it's unlikely, but indeed possible.

Because it is difficult to conceive while on your period, many women consider it a form of contraception. *But...* (you knew there'd be a "but," didn't you?) women who have shorter intervals between periods—say, twenty-one days or so, meaning that they ovulate on day *seven* or *eight*—may be prone to getting pregnant at the end of a long period!

Ovulation is the twenty-four-hour window when the egg is available for the sperm to fertilize. A woman having fewer days between periods would ovulate earlier in the month. That is why women with shorter period cycles can get pregnant with unprotected sex on an unexpected day.

Even though the risk of pregnancy is small, it is a possibility, especially when you consider that sperm can live for up to five days!

### *Douching After Sex as a Form of Birth Control*

Let me put it this way: Just say no to douching, anytime, anywhere, for cleaning or contraception.

Not only is douching a mythic form of birth control, it is a bad habit. Douches are premade cleansing mixtures that come in plastic bottles to be squirted high up into the vagina as a way of cleansing the vagina and helping it to smell fresh and clean. The truth is that douches neither cleanse nor act as contraception. In fact—as I pointed out earlier—the active cleaning ingredients used in most douches can upset the healthy vaginal discharge and pH balance of the vagina, thus resulting in a yeast or bacterial infection.

Really, there is never a reason to douche!

## *Breastfeeding Prevents Pregnancy*

Okay, so you're breastfeeding after the birth of your child—bravo! But, if you're thinking that you're guaranteed active contraception during the process, you may be sadly mistaken.

Most women do not think that it's possible to become pregnant during their postpartum recovery period. They believe, or have been told, that they can't get pregnant until their period returns. Unfortunately, this is just not the case. Ask anyone with "Irish twins"—a term referring to siblings born less than twelve months apart.

So, in fact, it's absolutely possible to get pregnant while breastfeeding, unless you happen to be following the birth control method of Lactational Amenorrhea Method (LAM) to a T. These guidelines for this particular birth control method include the following:

- Your nursing baby must be less than six months old.
- You must not have experienced a return of menstruation.
- You are taking no regular supplements.
- You are breastfeeding at least eight times in twenty-four hours, including night feedings.

If these guidelines are followed closely, your chances of pregnancy are less than 2 percent. Otherwise, if you're not practicing abstinence or safe sex, you may be surprised to find yourself pregnant while breastfeeding.

The reason for unplanned pregnancies while breastfeeding is simply this: most women believe they can't get pregnant during their postpartum recovery because they haven't resumed their period. But the truth is that if you haven't had a period after giving birth, you may indeed be starting to *ovulate*, since ovulation occurs *before* a period. And it is during ovulation that pregnancy occurs.

Statistics vary in revealing what percentage of women have become pregnant while breastfeeding—ranging from 5 to 28 percent and depending on whether the pregnancy occurred during the first six months postpartum or later. But one thing is certain; the further you are from giving birth, the greater the chance of getting pregnant if you are not using reliable contraception.

Obviously, with all the misinformation about breastfeeding as a birth control method floating around, there is a need for health care providers to educate women on birth control practices and pregnancy prevention during the standard six-week post-delivery visit, if not sooner!

### *Facts and Fallacies About the Pill*

I'm always surprised by the misinformation that continues to float around the birth control pill—a form of contraception that has been a godsend to many women since it was introduced in the 1960s.

Just to set the record straight, here are some of the top truths and arguments I have most often heard about the Pill:

* **It makes me fat!** It's true—to some extent. The Pill definitely has noticeable side effects during the initial two to three months of taking it. The most common of those effects are breakthrough or irregular bleeding, breast tenderness, nausea, bloating, and headache. You may experience one or more or none of these side effects when transitioning to this particular form of contraception, as well as a bit of weight gain as a result of fluid retention. The scale may show a one- to three-pound weight gain, but studies show that this is only a temporary side effect.

  A review of reliable medical literature shows no evidence of permanent weight gain in most women due to the Pill.

* **Smoking and The Pill.** If you do smoke—and you shouldn't be, but, if you do—and you are over the age of thirty-five, there are safety risks in taking The Pill. The hormones in the pill can make your blood thicker than usual, leading to hypercoagulation, which is the medical term for excessive clotting. With excessive clotting comes blood clots, which are jelly-like clumps of blood that may break free and travel through your veins to your heart and lungs, thus preventing blood flow.

  Women at high risk for blood clots include those using estrogen (birth control) and those who smoke. As we all know, smoking itself is a health risk, but smoking and the Pill are an even riskier combination.

  And while we're on the subject...

* **Blood Clots and The Pill.** If you already have a history of blood clots, the Pill is definitely not for you. When a clot develops and breaks free, it can travel to any number of places in your body. A pulmonary embolism refers to a clot that has traveled to your lungs, creating a life-threatening situation. A clot in your brain can lead to stroke. No matter the destination of a blood clot, the results are extremely dangerous, if not deadly.

  The Pill is not for you if clotting is already in your history, or even in the medical history of your family. Talk to your health care provider.

### *Facts and Fallacies About the IUD*

The contraceptive device known as an IUD—Intrauterine Device—is a small T-shaped flexible device that is inserted into the uterus in order to prevent pregnancy. Even more so than the Pill, it has had its share of bad raps, misinformation, and myth, which is why it's necessary to set the record straight on this stalwart device.

* **Ultimate Myth #1: The IUD is Not Recommended for Teens *or* Women Who Have Never Been Pregnant.** This is one of the most common bits of misinformation I've heard about IUDs. The fact is that, in a recent committee opinion on adolescents and Long Acting Reversible Contraceptions (LARCs), the American College of Obstetricians and Gynecologists (ACOG) *recommends the IUD as a "first line" option for all women of reproductive age.* After years of testing and observation, we now know that IUDs are safe for women, regardless of whether or not they have been pregnant.

In fact, there are certain types of IUDs that may work best for those who have never been pregnant, and therefore have smaller uterine cavities. The Skyla, Kyleena, and Liletta brands of IUDs may be best suited for that particular category of women.

Be assured, there is no reason not to choose the IUD, especially if convenience is your biggest concern.

* **The IUD Can Cause Infertility.** So, back in the old days—way back in the 1970s—the Dalkon Shield brand of IUD was found to cause pelvic infections in a disproportionally large percentage of users, resulting in infertility. It seems that a design flaw involving a bacteria-friendly string in the device led to those pelvic infections. Fortunately, lessons were learned by those early mistakes, and, after extensive studies on the safety and efficacy of the next generations of IUDs, the results were clear: The current IUDs—including Paragard, Mirena, Skylar, Kyleena, and Liletta—have been proven to be well-studied and completely safe.

  Your biggest risk factor for infertility? A previously undetected infection along the lines of chlamydia or gonorrhea. So, before you have that IUD inserted, have your health care provider screen you for STIs.

* **Insertion of the IUD is Difficult and/or Painful!** Depending on your pain tolerance, you might want to prep yourself thirty minutes before insertion of an IUD with 600 to 800 mg of ibuprofen. That is simply a suggestion, as many women tend to feel anything from a bit of cramping to a sharp pain during insertion—partly

due to the fact that the IUD must pass through your cervix in order to be situated inside your uterus.

However, I do believe there is a *best* time for an IUD insertion procedure, and that is immediately following your last period, as your cervix is more dilated during and right after your period.

While studies show that the IUD has made a serious comeback and tends to have the "highest patient satisfaction" amongst contraception users, there may be reasons why it's not best in *your* particular case. As with any mode of contraception, it is always a good idea to discuss your risks and benefits with your health care provider.

## Confusion Beyond the Vagina

Of course, as important and powerful as our vaginas are, women's health does extend beyond that unique and extraordinary organ. When it comes to breast health and concerns, I can be nearly as obsessive as I am regarding vaginas. So, before closing this chapter, I'd like to address just a few concerns that I most often hear in my own practice.

### *Is it Normal to Have Nipple Hair?*

Believe it or not, I get this question *a lot,* so here goes...

Certainly, there are some women who have never experienced a popup nipple hair—or two or three—but the truth is that, depending upon the stage of your life and hormonal surges, you most likely will develop some strays. And that is perfectly normal.

The area around the nipples, known as the areola, naturally has hair follicles. Puberty, pregnancy, and menopause are typically times in women's lives when hormonal changes are more physically noticeable, and those changes often include random hair growth wherever a follicle might be. Some women are more prone to this growth than others, but don't get too smug. It you've so far avoided the occasional nipple hairs, chances are that, if you start noticing random growths of hair on your chin and face, your nipple follicles may take the cue.

### *What is Nipple Discharge? And is it Normal?*

Women *expect* nipple discharge during pregnancy but tend to be concerned if they experience it outside of a pregnancy. Don't worry. Nipple discharge can be a very normal occurrence for women who are not anywhere near pregnant.

Clear fluid from the nipples can result from excess stimulation during intimacy, sex, or exercise. Tight T-shirts or bras may also cause leakage during exercise from rubbing the nipples. Also, drugs such as birth control pills, thyroid, and psychiatric medications may cause nipple discharge.

If you're at all worried, or if the discharge is excessive or it's a strange color or is accompanied by pain or a lump in the breast, then I would recommend you consult with your health care provider. But rarely is nipple discharge a sign of cancer.

### *Are Breast Lumps Always a Cause for Concern?*

Breast lumps are common—affecting eight out of ten women—and, fortunately, most are *not* cancerous. Depending upon where in your menstrual cycle you are, you will probably detect some lumps. Chances are, if you feel a breast lump just prior to your period, it will disappear by your period's end.

During the premenstrual time, hormones can cause an increase in the nodularity of breast tissue—simply meaning a greater tendency for small lumps and nodules. This nodularity tends to create benign cysts, the kind that ultimately go away. However, if you have a persistent breast lump, it is important to have your doctor examine you in order to determine if testing, such as breast ultrasound, is necessary.

In the instance of breast lumps (as with other things) size does not matter—big or small, a breast lump that does not go away should be properly evaluated.

### *Why Does One Breast Always Seem to be Bigger?*

As no two snowflakes (or bodies, or ears, or lips, or vaginas!) are alike, no two breasts—no matter if they're of a *pair*—are alike. One breast will always, to some degree, seem of a different size than the other, and that is completely normal. Different *is* normal.

### *When Do I Start Going for Mammograms? And How Often?*

You probably already know the statistics: One in eight women will develop breast cancer in their lifetime. To that effect, more women than ever are aware of the need for breast cancer screening. Unfortunately, as awareness has increased, the issue of the whens, whys, and hows of cancer screenings have become more complicated as well. Physicians and patients are equally confused as to which guidelines to follow, as different medical organizations have different recommendations.

The current guidelines issued by the American College of Obstetricians/Gynecologists recommend starting mammogram screening at age forty, with regular screenings once every one to two years, increasing to yearly at age fifty. However, the American Cancer Society recommends annual screenings starting at age forty-five, with follow-ups every other year until age fifty-five (at which point, screenings should be done yearly).

The one factor that both reputable organizations can agree upon is that every woman needs to know her own individual risk factors for the disease.

Those risk factors for breast cancer include:

* Number of first-degree relatives with breast cancer
* Onset of puberty (menstrual period) before age twelve
* First pregnancy after age thirty
* No full-term pregnancy
* Number of previous biopsies
* Personal history of breast cancer
* Presence of atypical hyperplasia—a precancerous condition of breast cells
* Mammographic breast density
* Excessive alcohol consumption
* BMI greater than 30
* Physical inactivity

No matter when you start, a mammogram is the only cost-effective screening available for early detection of breast cancer, and a best weapon in reducing the risk of death from breast cancer. However, if you know you are at a high risk, or you simply want a more thorough screening for breast cancer, you may want to opt for a 3-D mammogram as it combines multiple breast X-ray images to create a 3-D image of the breast. This particular screening, as well as being able to identify more cancers than a regular 2-D mammogram, has a 40 percent less chance of providing false positive results.

Not all screening facilities offer 3-D mammograms, and not all insurance companies will cover them. Check with your health care provider to discuss your options.

Become actively involved in your breast health. Know your personal risk factors. Make informed decisions and be the champion of *your girls*.

Bottom line: Know your female anatomy from head to toe. Be aware of all the miraculous things you and your body are capable of, and understand the care and maintenance that body requires. Take the initiative in your self-knowledge, as that knowledge is your best defense against misunderstanding the subtle (and not so subtle) signals your body may send you. I don't want you to ever be scratching your head—or your labia—in confusion about what is normal or not. And, when in doubt, consult a trusted health care provider.

Your health—your *female* health, your *whole* health, body and mind—no matter the chapter of your life, is your responsibility, not only to yourself, but also to the people you love. Take an active role in your health care and the *prevention* of illness and disease. Treat yourself, *care* for yourself, as you would your most cherished family member, friend, or lover because you owe it to yourself and to them.

Speak up. Ask questions. Demand transparency in the care you receive. It is my hope that *She-ology* and I can help you be your own best and informed advocate on whatever journey you may be.

Thank you for joining me in changing the narrative on how we talk about women's health and sexuality. Now, let's continue the important conversations about our Lady Parts!

With love and appreciation,

*—Dr. Sherry*

# ABOUT SHE-OLOGY

## Hormonal Products and Relatable Medical Information for Women

Along my journey in writing *She-ology* and *She-ology, the Shequel,* I had the opportunity to do extensive research on the latest trends, opinions, and concerns of women all over the country. In doing so, I realized that the narrative on female health was greatly in need of improvement.

I found that women were eager to discuss sensitive issues of body and mind, and that, more often than not, these issues centered around trying to manage the symptoms and effects of the *normal* hormonal cycles of PMS, perimenopause, menopause, puberty, infertility, pregnancy, and postpartum. Specifically, women wanted healthy and safe alternatives to prescription medication in order to manage those hormonal cycles. I realized there was a need for innovative health supplements designed specifically for women in order for them to feel their very best during each specific cycle.

To meet that need, I was fortunate enough to partner with Coast Science in creating supplements formulated especially for women with safe, healthy, and clinically-proven ingredients to support normal hormonal cycles. This collaboration with Coast Science led to the *online site* She-ology, where women can go to continue the conversation with me about their health concerns, as well as find scientifically-researched supplements to address their specific hormonal needs.

*Vive la différence!*

# ACKNOWLEDGMENTS

I am not going to lie. This has been the most challenging year of my life. The death of my ever dynamic, seemingly invincible father from pancreatic cancer in November 2018 brought the lives of my family and me to a complete standstill.

As my father lay in bed that last week of his life—and although he was too weak for most conversation—his sense of humor and acute awareness of the world around him remained intact. I read him my Leaky V chapter, because I imagined that he, as a retired urologist, might have one last bit of advice for me. Although he loved to tease me with his doctor's humor by telling me that "gynecologists had nothing over urologists when it came to urinary incontinence," he did, in fact, give me one last approving smile, meaning that my content was, indeed, accurate.

My father taught me to find my passion and to reach for the stars. Often in my life, I heard him say, "If you throw enough shit against the wall, something will stick." That edict has translated into my throwing my heart into changing the narrative on how women talk about their bodies and their vaginas. It means that, as long as I have a voice, I will carry on the conversation on women's health and happiness and education. It has been in doing so that I felt the need to write this second book.

Mom, thank you for your unwavering support of everything I do—and for your memories of how, throughout my childhood, I would write in my journal late at night, "en route to becoming an author." As with so many of my endeavors, you knew before I did that I had the ability to succeed, and you championed me when I needed it the most. I feel your hand in everything I do. Not a day that goes by that I don't appreciate how fortunate I am to have you as my mother, my best friend, and my inspiration.

To my patients: Seriously, where would I be without you? I believe I learn as much from you as you profess to learn from me. Your support, encouragement, and joyful participation in my she-quel have touched me profoundly. I hope I've done justice to your input and advice. A special thanks to Lisa Hide Ross, Elyse Reisch, and those who were brave enough to share their most personal stories with my readers.

To those friends who helped add a special dimension to *She-ology*: Jennifer Beals, Holly Coombs, Zooey Deschanel, Kym Douglas, Kirsten Dunst, Sara Foster, Shenae Grimes-Beech, Eileen Kelly, Kiki Melendez, Kevin Nealon, Paula Pell, Rachel Roberts, Camila Sodi, Elizabeth Turner, Sela Ward, and Suzanne Westenhoefer, it has been an honor to share in the intimate times of your lives—times that have been both wondrous and difficult. I am so grateful for your contributions.

To Julia Ormond, special thanks for your inspired and enlightening introduction. Your honesty and authenticity are a breath of fresh air, always.

To those women who have stood arm in arm, in support of me and my crazy dreams: Karen Rizzo, you are a wordsmith—I could not have chosen a better writing partner. Danielle "Dani" Tatum, my badass nurse, your dedication and sense of humor make it possible for me to squeeze twenty-five hours out of every workday. Harriet Sternberg, my advisor extraordinaire,

I thank you for supporting and believing in me through all these years of our cherished friendship.

Ana “Magumi” Wade, thank you, again, for lending your artistic talents in bringing my chapters to life. With any luck, your anthropomorphic vaginas will one day have their own animated series!

To my dream posse that helps elevate me in all my projects, my best friends and sisters, Brenda Daly, Jennifer Brown, Johanna Daly, Debbie Battaglia, Mary Connelly, Julie Silver, Veronica Gutierrez, Susannah Gutierrez, Polita Gutierrez, Allison Enciso, Mel Silvernail, and The Wolfe Pack (!): How is it that I am so blessed to have your love and support? I don’t know where I would be without our family dinners and all of you on speed dial for those late night and wee-hour-of-the-morning calls.

Nena Medonia, your belief in my ability to write these books, as well as your encouragement and kindness, have been a gift all along this journey.

To my sons, Michael, Stephen, and Jonathan Becker: I am so blessed to have such compassionate, conscious, and loving young men as you three in my life. Your obvious respect for women, the environment, and family is my biggest source of pride. You are the best of what men can be.

Finally, to my wife and partner in love and life, Peggy Gutierrez: Thank you for supporting me and allowing me to chase my dreams. Your patience and unconditional love energize and inspire me daily. With you by my side, there is nothing I can’t do, forever and ever is never enough for me!

# ABOUT THE AUTHOR

Sheryl A. Ross, M.D.—known as "Dr. Sherry" by her patients—is an award-winning OB/GYN, author, entrepreneur, and women's health expert. In her nearly thirty years of practice, Dr. Sherry has received numerous ongoing awards and honors including the Patient's Choice Award for Compassionate Doctor Recognition and Southern California Super Doctor. Castle Connolly named her as a Top Doctor and Exceptional Woman in Obstetrics & Gynecology.

Dr. Sherry recently received the Angel Award for being a physician outstanding in her field who has made a significant contribution as a role model to women everywhere.

Dr. Sherry is the founder of She-ology: a first-of-its-kind women's wellness brand to create female-focused supplements to support hormonal changes experienced by women. Dr. Sherry created the She-ology award-winning five-piece wearable vaginal dilator set designed with your active lifestyle in mind to stretch the vaginal opening, restore vaginal capacity by expanding the vagina in width and depth, and help users resume comfortable and more enjoyable sexual intercourse or self-stimulation. Dr. Sherry is also the co-founder of the Heartlanta Bra—uniquely designed for women's bodies during stress echocardiogram tests. She is also a spokesperson ambassador for the American Heart Association and GoRed supporting women and heart disease.

Dr. Sherry was a medical consultant for the books, *Expecting Fitness* and *Two at a Time*. She is featured in the *HuffPost,*

*Marie Claire, Cosmo,* Yahoo, *Redbook, Teen Vogue,* Fox News, *Glamour, Bustle,* WebMD, *Redbook, Readers Digest,* Medscape, and many more. Dr. Sherry has made TV appearances on *Good Morning America, Rachel Ray, Pickler & Ben, Home & Family,* and *Inside Edition*—just to name a few.

In addition to her medical practice, Dr. Sherry is on the board of Planned Parenthood in Los Angeles. You can connect with Dr. Sherry and learn more about She-ology by visiting www.DrSherry.com and www.She-ology.com. She also shares her knowledge with others on Twitter @DrSherylRoss, Instagram @drsherryr and on Facebook DrSherryR.

# ABOUT THE ILLUSTRATOR

Ann-Marisa Wada is a painter and illustrator. She is also a high school visual arts teacher at Alain Leroy Locke College Prep Academy in Watts, California.

She was born and raised in Santa Monica, California. In 1999, she and her family moved to Tokyo, Japan, where she graduated from an international high school and went on to graduate from Temple University Japan and Tyler School of Art. She received a Master's in Education from Loyola Marymount University.

Dr. Sherry Ross M.D featured Ann-Marisa's illustrations in the first *She-ology*.

Personal Art Instagram: @mdub_art

Art Teaching Instagram: @mdub_studioz

## Also by Sherry A. Ross, MD

*She-ology:*
*The Definitive Guide to*
*Women's Intimate Health. Period.*